WHY ME?

My Journey from M.E. to Health and Happiness

Updated Edition 2014

Alex Howard

First edition published 2003, second edition published 2009 and this third edition published 2014 by Cherry Red Books, a division of Cherry Red Records, Power Road Studios, W4 5PY, London
Copyright © 2003, 2009, 2014 Alex Howard

Typeset by Sarah Reed.
Cover Design by Jim Phelan at Wolf Graphics.
Photos by Abigail Zoe Martin.

ISBN 978-1-909454-19-4

www.FreedomFromME.co.uk

Acknowledgements

Sitting here thinking of those who have impacted on my life, I am filled with the deepest gratitude. Of all those who assisted in my journey, there is one person without whom this book would never have been written: my uncle Iain McNay. The impact he has had on my life will be obvious to everyone who shares my journey.

There have been many teachers along my path who have impacted on my journey in some way, and I've recommended books at the end of those whose work I encourage you to explore.

Those who have helped in proof reading, and assisted me in clarifying my ideas in writing, are Catherine Buchan, Diane Fenton, Ashley Meyer, Penny Faith, Gabrielle Wellington-Spurr and Alison Manos. For the second and third editions, I'd also like to thank Anna Duschinsky, Val Duschinsky, Anna King and Richard Anderson for their suggestions and editing.

I would also like to express a public thank you to The Optimum Health Clinic team. Your tireless work and commitment has made so many things possible. It is because of your determination, integrity and endless dedication that we've been able to help so many people in so many difficult situations. May our shared vision continue to blossom and flourish as we continue to spread the word that recovery really is possible.

Finally, to my wife and beloved, Tania and our two beautiful daughters Marli and Ariella, you make every day a blessing and those years of suffering worth it in every way.

FOREWORD
By Shirley Conran OBE

It is said that everyone has a book in them. This is not true: some people don't have even a paragraph. However, Alex Howard is a walking library: first there's the story of Man battling against Adversity, then Man on a Quest, followed by a Medical Detective and finally Love Story with Happy Ending when two people part.

I always want to know what happened after the end of a book, particularly so when, some years ago, I read Alex Howard's WHY ME? because Alex and I have something in common: M.E.

Forty years ago, when I was Woman's Editor of the Daily Mail, I went into hospital with viral pneumonia and came out with M.E., to face a wall of medical disbelief that I was ill. My GP sent me to three different "experts"; quickly, I realised that they were psychiatrists, quickly I realised that they were wrong in their diagnoses: I am not workshy, I do not need to draw attention to myself and I am not a hypochondriac. Quickly I realised that the medical profession was saying, "If we cannot find anything physically wrong with you, then you must be mad, to some degree." When I realised that it was the medical profession that was wrong, I decided to avoid their Kafkaesque attitudes and deal by myself with the symptoms of my illness.

However, when every medical expert is telling you that black is white, when your family is worried about your odd behaviour, and when you lose your job and your income, you probably will need a psychiatrist. Eventually I met one, who said, "I'm going to assume that everything you say is true". He understood my contempt for psychiatrists and from then on, he helped me deal with my symptoms. Once he scribbled a note to my new GP. "What have you told him?" I snapped. He took the note out of the envelope and handed it to me. It read, "Dear Colleague, contrary to what you may at first believe, this patient tells the truth. Yours sincerely, Jonathan Gould". So he meant what he had said, when first we met.

One day my mother said, "You've changed for the better, since you met that Dr Gould". Certainly, I had stopped being an appeasing, unctuous, eyelash-batting, role-playing little woman. Now, I didn't care what people thought of me, but what I thought of those people; now I stood up for my own opinions; I became friendly with my body; I learned to be my true self. I grew up.

Eventually, I no longer had money problems: I could afford to have M.E. because I made a fortune in property and another fortune when I became an international author. I travelled round the world eight times, seven of those at the expense of my publishers. I was able to financially help my children when they needed it.

One day I realised that the silver lining of M.E. is that it pushes you onto your own resources; it forces you to think for yourself and to create your own disciplines and determination, because the only person that can understand your condition and improve it …is YOU.

Dr Gould died and for the next twenty years I spent a fortune trying everything that claimed to cure or help M.E. None of it worked.

Then I read a book and immediately identified with the young author, who had been bedridden for two years as a teenager. Alex Howard eventually earned a first class degree in psychology and Swansea University should be proud of him.

"WHY ME?" was a gangly, exuberant book and the dynamism and determination of the author shone beyond the grammatical errors (I'm still an editor!). Three years ago, I actually met Alex. Meeting someone with M.E, forced to lead a similar life to yours, is like meeting someone who comes from your home town and speaks your language, after you have spent years in a foreign land. Because Alex had dealt so successfully with his illness - and was clearly helping others to do so - I decided to ask for his help. So Alex became my mentor. We talk for an hour every fortnight. My health and my well being have improved considerably.

Often when a new edition of a book is published, it adds nothing much of value. But, the added chapters of WHY ME? kept me up beyond midnight, and I used the highlighter so much that some pages are almost yellow.

Alex takes the reader along his journey through adversity to success; he does not hesitate to tell of his stupid behaviour: he succumbed to the temptation of overworking and he suffered the consequences. He struggled financially and emotionally to reach his well-deserved success, both personally and with his clinic The Optimum Health Clinic.

In this new edition, the autobiographical sequence - what Alex did next - is followed by three transcripts of TV interviews with the three directors of The Optimum Health Clinic. And - to use two of Alex's favourite adjectives - these chapters are incredibly amazing.

I shall re-read them tonight, and often afterwards, because - to my surprise - just reading these added chapters has taken me a step further in my own M.E. quest for health. I nearly wrote "battle with M.E.", but I no longer regard M.E. as my enemy. I look upon my symptoms as messages from my body that I reached burnout in the past because of my determined, stressful, body-ignoring behaviour. I now suspect that my M.E. is partly the result of living a hardworking, exciting, adrenal-filled life in a way that my body could no longer tolerate, but that I refused to face.

For three years, I have argued with Alex that complete recovery in M.E. is not possible.

Now, I am not so sure.

Having read this new edition of "WHY ME?" I have a new courage, a new willingness to explore where I have - until now - refused to go. I have a new optimism based on facts that I know are scientifically proven, not some mindless, new, fix-fast "discipline". My determination has been renewed. I feel that I have just started to take the next step towards… dare I say it…recovery. I wish you the same good fortune.

Shirley Conran OBE
London, August 2009

Introduction To Third Edition

It is now over eleven years since I finished working on the first edition of this book. One third of my life. In that time so much has happened. The seven-year period you are about to read about in many ways feels like a distant memory. On one hand it is hard for me to see the world through the eyes of that terrified boy who woke up one morning to face his world falling apart. On the other hand, in my work with The Optimum Health Clinic I am reminded almost daily of the fear, loneliness and pain we experience when battling with an illness like ME/CFS. For me, the personal suffering is over, but for you, the journey may just be beginning. If so, I hope in some way this book can be a companion and guide for you.

Reading back through some of these pages with the benefit of the last eleven years is an odd experience. I hear a younger voice to the one I know of myself now. A voice that is at times perhaps a little righteous, and at others utterly indignant of those who I felt should have helped me and didn't. With the perspectives that come from over a decade working as a professional in the field, I feel a little more considered in my opinions, yet I also realise my younger voice is as important now as it was then.

Yes, there are many complex reasons why conventionally available treatments for ME/CFS are decades behind those being pioneered in clinics such as The Optimum Health Clinic. There are many well-intentioned people simply working with fundamentally flawed ideas, but things are slowly changing. We can seek to understand, we can be compassionate and we can cultivate patience.

But, for the sixteen year old me that woke up to a life destroyed, and the eighteen year old me that considered taking his life, I will not soften my words or attempt to be more politically correct. When I found my path out of ME/CFS, I wanted to scream it from the rooftops and shove it down the throats of all those who had failed in their duty to help. And, I had every right to feel that way.

Treatment of ME/CFS in this country is a scandal - hundreds of thousands of people in the UK alone suffer from an illness that has clear causes, effective treatments, and identifiable biomarkers. They're generally either told it is all in their heads and there is nothing wrong with them, or that they're seriously chronically ill and they will never recover. This is not good enough - in my day job it is appropriate I choose my words carefully when speaking publicly, but here I will not censor myself. People with ME/CFS deserve better. You deserve better. Things need to change, and it can start with you and I.

Here is my story. One day I hope to hear yours.

Alex Howard
London, July 2014

Introduction

These are mediocre times.
People are starting to lose hope.
It's hard for many to believe there are extraordinary things inside
themselves and others.
I hope you can keep an open mind.
Unbreakable

As a child I always loved stories of great adventure and discovery. Films such as Star Wars, Back to the Future and The Karate Kid consistently held a special place in my heart. I often dreamed about experiencing my own quest and story of dramatic transformation. Along the way I would meet wise teachers who would teach me great things, towards the end I would fall in love, and there would then be a dramatic climax where I did great things. Yet, by the age of fifteen years old I had all but given up hope of my quest, telling myself that such adventures only happened to other people. I was wrong. My own quest did happen, but it started in the least likely of places and the most surprising of ways

One day I woke up and something in me was different. I was very seriously ill, but no one had any idea what I was actually ill with. In time it became apparent that I had developed one of the most poorly misunderstood chronic illnesses known in Western society, an illness for which according to the world's "experts" there is no cure. "Why have I got ME? Why is this happening to me?" I endlessly questioned as I spent several years virtually bed-bound and sinking into a deeper and deeper clinical depression. Then, one day someone planted a seed of belief in my mind that just perhaps I did have all I needed to transform my life and my world, regardless of what traditional thinking suggested. Feeling like I had no other choice, I gave every ounce of my desperate existence to finding a cure for my ME, along with my clinical depression and major anxiety.

When I consider my world these days I still ask, "Why me?" but I ask from a very different place. Why was I able to change something that is apparently unchangeable? Why do I now have a quality of life that seven years ago I could only have dreamed of being possible? You hold the answers to these questions in your hands. I pray that as you let them sink into your heart they will be more than just intellectual concepts. Knowledge is nice. Action creates change.

In love and warmth,
Alex Howard,

Contents

*Dedicated to all those I have been fortunate
enough to work with over the years.*

*Your desire to create change in the face of often seemingly
insurmountable adversity inspires me every day.*

Alex will be donating all royalties from this edition of "WHY ME?" to registered charity The Optimum Health Clinic Foundation. The Optimum Health Clinic was founded by Alex in 2004, with a commitment to make integrative medicine treatment for ME/CFS available to all. The Optimum Health Clinic is currently working on a randomised controlled trial as a key step towards one day hopefully government funding being available for treatment.

Registered Charity number 1131664

CHAPTER 1: A NIGHT OF CELEBRATION (SUMMER 1996)

Your vision will only become clear when you look inside of your own heart.
Who looks outside, dreams.
Who looks inside, awakens.
Carl Jung

It was the perfect summer evening. The hot sun of the day was slowly draining away and leaving a gentle warmth. My girlfriend Emily and I were on our way to some friends after spending a relaxing day together enjoying the growing anticipation of three months of freedom. We were both nearing the end of our GCSE's and only had a couple of exams left. There was a magical feeling of passion between us. It was like one plus one equalled ten when we were together. Emily had shoulder length blonde hair and a good figure; I was hoping that in the near future I was going to be exposed to more of her beauty.

I had fancied Emily throughout most of secondary school, but by the last year I had given up hope. I had been genuinely surprised when she had asked me out in the last few weeks of term. Much to my mum and stepfather's frustration, we spoke on the telephone every night, despite usually having seen each other in the day. The telephone bills were a stretch for them to pay, but I didn't care; I felt as if I was falling in love for the first time.

We got a lift from Emily's parents over to her cousin's beautiful house in the Surrey countryside. It had five or six bedrooms and acres of land, very different to where I lived. Our friends were already there and soon we were lost in conversation, me with the guys and Emily with the girls. Apart from hoping to make use of the empty house with Emily and beat my mates in the race to lose our virginity, I was also particularly excited about talking to Tom, Dale and Nick about the band we were starting on Friday.

As the four of us sat round a table swigging our cans of beer, which we had stolen from our parents, we got planning.

"We can use my basement to jam," offered Nick, our newly discovered drummer, as he opened another can of beer.

"Cool man," said Tom, our singer, in his slow, deep voice. "I've got a few new riffs we can jam on." Tom was one of the more trendy guys at school, and I was loving the fact that I was now associated with such people.

"I'm gonna borrow a bass guitar from a guy my dad knows," added Dale, one of my closest friends, as he crushed an empty can in his hand.

1

"Wicked," I said, trying to sound as cool as I could. "I have a few new tunes as well, I've also worked out the guitar solo to that Ash song 'Uncle Pat.' Sounds well good."
"No way," said Tom, tossing his hair out of his eyes, "That's a bitching solo, I can't wait to hear it."

And so we continued together, plotting our path to international stardom. After a while Emily caught my eye and I left the guys to spend some time with her.

As the golden sun continued to go down over the rolling Surrey hills, Emily and I headed for a walk alone together in the woods. While we strolled along side by side, hand in hand, my mind drifted back to the events of the recent months. I had scored reasonable grades in my mock exams the previous Christmas, but there were very high expectations in my family. My two elder cousins and sister, Georgina, had set the standard by achieving twenty-seven A's and only three B's between them. Such expectations led to a fair amount of pressure on me. Of course I was assured that it was the kind of person I was that mattered. However, children are sensitive to their environment, and years of torment from both family and peers told me different.

The coming months were to see some exciting changes in my life. It was really starting to feel like the traumas of the past were over and I could finally forget about the horrors that had made up my family life. The attempted suicides, the violence, the abuse and the alcoholism, perhaps they were all finally done with? I wanted to look forward, not back, for I had always believed that was where my happiness lay.

Emily and I carried on walking and reached a rubber tyre hanging from an old oak tree. We took it in turns to sit on the tyre and gently push each other. As I caught the swing and pushed her again, we caught each other's eye.
"You seem a bit quiet," Emily said to me inquisitively, " Are you okay?"
"Yeah I'm fine," I replied, "I'm just glad to be getting away from Ashcombe. You know what I went through at that school. I can't wait to start the band on Friday. I really think we're gonna rock."

Soon we got bored with the swing and sat down in the grass nearby. I leant forward and kissed Emily's neck, working up towards her mouth. Putting my arms around her I gently stroked her back, not daring to let my hands rove where I really wanted them to. It was a strange situation: I knew what I wanted, but I had such mixed feelings about going for it. What if Emily wasn't ready? What if I ruined what we had? Perhaps even more frightening, what if she actually did want to as well? Of course talking about the idea was out of the question. Such a conversation was not in our dialogue.

After some more kissing and cuddling, and my guessing that the issue had been avoided for another day, we made our way back to the house and rejoined the celebrations. I was starting to feel less carefree. I was going to have to go home soon. My mum and stepfather didn't trust me enough to let me stay the night. This meant I was going to have to leave the party just as it started to reach its climax. This annoyed me, as did most things to do with my family.

As I waited for the embarrassment of being picked up at 11:00, Emily made my heart stop.
"I'm so drunk I would probably sleep with you," she whispered in my ear.
Wow, I thought to myself, she does want it too! My mind started to imagine one of my wildest dreams coming true: having sex with the girl I had fancied consistently for four years. At this point, I didn't even care about the fact that I would be beating most of my friends to it. It was a precious moment. Even I knew it.

However, despite the fact that I was a rather intoxicated teenager with raging hormones, my conscience told me to be cautious. If Emily really was drunk, then maybe she might regret it the following morning? If she needed alcohol to be ready, did that not mean she needed more time? I knew what I wanted, but I also cared about her. Surely one more night of chastity was worth it, just to make sure, I reasoned. After all, the summer was mine to do with as I pleased. There would be plenty of other chances.
"I have to go soon," was the best excuse I could come up with. The light was poor and I never saw the reaction in Emily's face as a group of friends joined us. The beauty of the moment disappeared as fast as it had emerged. One thing was for sure though: my life was going from good to great.

While I waited for my mum and stepfather to arrive, my friends and I sat around chatting about the last four years of school and our plans for the future. Most people, like Emily, were just going to start a course that interested them and see where they ended up. Tom, Dale and Nick were all in this category, they thought playing music was "cool and everything," but they didn't really believe we could make it in the music industry. Dale probably came closest to sharing my drive and ambition, but even for him success was more of a nice idea than a necessity. It was different for me. I needed to do something special with my life. I wanted more and I wasn't scared to ask for it. I hated the world I had grown up in and I was willing to do whatever it took to avoid that kind of life.

As I sat in the car with my mum and stepfather on the way home half an hour later, I made my frustration at having to leave early known by ignoring them. This was a progression from mumbling my words and slouching my shoulders when I was only mildly annoyed with them. When we arrived home, I went straight to my room and rolled out my dumbbells from under my bed. I used my angst at my family to help me lift my weights in my intoxicated state. I reasoned that to be a successful musician I had to look the part. Despite the fact that I had been lifting weights for several months with no obvious difference, I still kept at it every day without fail.

Getting into bed that night I was the happiest I could remember being. Two of the most exciting things that I could imagine were on my mind: Emily and I were going to have sex, and the guys and I were on our way to becoming famous. With the summer holidays also just about to start, I couldn't wait to get started. For the first time in my life I really felt like my dreams were coming true.

Turning over and falling asleep, my mind was overflowing with plans for the future.

That was to be my last night of health for years.

CHAPTER 2: THE MORNING AFTER

***Waking up sometimes needs a very loud alarm clock, especially if
we don't know we are sleeping.***

The estate where I grew up was several miles from the nearest town,
Dorking. The bus service was quite infrequent, and so the easiest way
to get there was to have a lift from Mum on her way to work. This
morning I had a hairdresser's appointment and so Mum woke me up at
8:00, ready to leave with her at 9:00. After the hairdressers, I had to go
and clean out one of the sheds at my grandparents' house in the middle
of Dorking. I didn't feel right. I couldn't put my finger on it. It wasn't
like a cold, I didn't ache, and I didn't feel sick. I somehow just didn't
feel right. I wondered if maybe I had a hangover. It seemed like the
only explanation, because I felt a bit like I was drunk, although it
wasn't quite the same. Whatever was wrong though, I just tried to
ignore it. I had to get to the hairdressers for my appointment; I wasn't
willing to hang around on my holidays.

Having gone through my morning routine of having a shower,
getting dressed, eating breakfast and cleaning my teeth, I managed to
get to the salon. As I sat in the chair I explained to my hairdresser,
Tony, that the same short back and sides as last time would be great.
Once he had started cutting, the conversation soon graduated towards
small talk. We discussed family, exams, the weather, and so on. I felt
like hell. My heartbeat was starting to feel like an accelerating train.
Even worse, with every faster beat my temperature was rising. It
seemed like it would only be a matter of time before I reached breaking
point, though I had no idea what that was. As my anxiety started to rise
in union with my heart rate and temperature, I tried to focus on what
was happening around me, attempting to take my mind off my body
and the storm I could feel brewing inside. It wasn't working.

Tony had been cutting my hair since I was a baby. It didn't feel like
that long since I had been coming for haircuts without my grandmother
accompanying me. Only a few months' ago I had had to work hard to
convince Tony to give me extremely short hair, so concerned was he
about the wrath of my family. Of course that only made me more
determined to have my hair cut shorter on future occasions.

The salon had the unforgettable smell of cut hair and hairspray, and
as it was the beginning of summer, it was quite busy. As I looked at
the locks of hair falling to the floor beside me, I wondered what would
happen to them. Would all those months of growth just be thrown
away?

The cutting continued. I really didn't feel right. My mind started telling me that I should say something, but what? I knew that explaining my situation would be very embarrassing, and could also land me in a fair amount of trouble when I got home. Drinking under age would not have been a problem, for I had been one of the few of my friends that didn't have to steal alcohol. My family was more than comfortable with drinking. However, letting this be known in public would be unacceptable.

I reasoned that it was too late now to do anything anyway. Tony had already taken large chunks of hair off the back of my head with the clippers. I could hardly go home with massive patches of hair missing. Maybe, I would be okay if I could just relax and not think about how I felt? Yes, that ought to work; you hear about how people get themselves into a panic and make things worse, I thought to myself. But I was a levelheaded person, and certainly had no history of panic attacks. Why would I start now? But why the hell couldn't I focus on the mirror in front of me? My heart was now going into palpitations; I was going to have to say something. I began to pass out. What was happening to me? What was wrong?

"Could I, erm, have a glass of water," I managed to mumble.

God, that sounded stupid, I attacked myself. Maybe it would help though; at least it would let Tony know that something was wrong.

"Sure, are you alright?" Tony asked, a slightly concerned expression on his face.

"Just feeling a bit dizzy," I managed to add, trying to smile to reassure him.

Tony walked off to get me some water and I struggled to pull myself together. However, the longer I sat there, the more nauseous I felt. The more nauseous I felt, the more scared I became. Unable to even influence what was happening in my own body, I started to develop more and more of a sense of helpless. I so wanted to tell someone how I really felt. But what could they do anyway? I certainly didn't want a scene. I decided that I would have to sit it out. If I fainted then at least I wouldn't have to battle anymore. Until something like that happened it seemed easier to say nothing.

The next thing I saw was the inside of a blurry ambulance, with a panicking paramedic rushing around beside me searching for something. Then my consciousness drifted off again and I was aware of lying in a hospital bed unable to speak. Everything was swirling into a daze in the whirlpool that had become my mind. Nothing seemed real. I felt like I didn't even exist. The only thing I knew was real was the fear that was burning inside.

Tony returned with a glass of water, and for a few seconds I remembered again that I was in the hairdressers. At least one of the assistants probably now knew there was something wrong, for they appeared to have been chatting in the next room. Maybe that was good, but maybe it also meant I was going to have to explain myself when I got home. That was hardly of much concern at the moment though. The only thing that really mattered right now was getting through the next ten minutes; getting my hair cut without falling apart. Then I could force myself home and get what was left of my head together.

Somehow, after being close to passing out another three or four times, I managed to survive the rest of the appointment giving relatively little away. Looking back, it seems obvious that I should have said something. After all, it was hardly my fault that I felt ill. But, at the time, that seemed impossible. Even my most basic senses of reasoning had left me. Hairdressing appointments were to haunt me for many years to come.

I decided to take a longer route to my grandparents' house, which was really only five minutes away, in the hope that I might be able to walk off whatever was wrong with me. It didn't work. However, it did help me to reduce some of the horrible tension I could feel inside. I wished that I didn't have to go and help out, but I felt like I had no proper excuse. The only explanation I had so far was that I had a hangover. That would certainly not be good enough. I didn't feel especially like resting anyway. I couldn't conceive of anything that would change the way that I felt apart from time, and I wanted to keep as busy as I could in that time. The last thing I wanted was to be alone with the cauldron of fear that had become my mind. I was meeting Emily later that afternoon and so I tried as hard as I could to focus on that.

Once I arrived at my grandparents, I briefly said "hello" before getting to work in the shed. I just wanted to get it finished. I knew that the sooner it was done, the sooner I would be able to leave. I have little memory of the next few hours, just intermittent recollections of a spinning dark hut, dusty flowerpots, and dozens and dozens of insects. Apparently I did manage to clear out the shed, sort out the flowerpots, and also have lunch. I have absolutely no recollection of eating at all.

That afternoon I confessed to Emily how strange I felt. She, too, thought it unlikely that I had a hangover. Nonetheless, she agreed it might be a good idea to go for another walk and get some fresh air. We therefore walked a couple of miles together in the hills at the back of where she lived. It had little effect. Her comment of the previous night was apparently forgotten. Sex was hardly top of my priorities anymore anyway; I was far too concerned with my current struggle with my mind and body. I also doubted Emily would even remember what she had said. She herself had admitted she was quite drunk. I assumed I would be feeling fine again soon and another opportunity would present itself.

The next day was band practice and Tom, Dale, Nick and I spent the day living out our fantasies of being rockstars. We climbed on the drum kit while playing, screamed lyrics at the tops of our voices, and thrashed our guitars and bashed the drums as fast and as hard as we could. There was, of course, also the making of the obligatory demo tape to play to our friends. As far as we were concerned, we were the best band in the world and we couldn't wait to prove it. First stop Nick's basement; next stop Wembley Stadium.

However, despite the adrenaline of my passion, there were several times in the day when the dizziness rose past a level that I felt I could cope with and I had to sit down. My head just didn't feel like it was properly attached to my shoulders. Every time I moved it seemed to want to fall off. As hard as I tried, I just couldn't seem to pull myself together.

The next morning I still felt like there was something very wrong with my balance, but I was less anxious about how I felt. I continued to assume that I would start to feel better soon. Resting didn't seem to make any difference, and so I decided that the best strategy would be to take it relatively easy, but for the most part try and get on with life as best I could.

My best friend, James, and I arranged to play golf together. James was, like me, around six feet tall and well built. He had shoulder length black hair and dark eyes. The two of us had spent most of the last year racing to grow our hair, as was the fashion amongst our friends. However, mine had just curled upwards and so I had eventually given up and had a French crop. James had been unable to make the party, as his final exam had been the day after. "Lucky git," I had thought to myself at the time. I was now rather pleased that I had more time until my last two. It would have been a nightmare to take an exam feeling the way I was.

James and I had been to different primary schools, but ever since discovering in our first year at secondary school that we both played golf we had spent almost every weekend together at the local golf club. It was a strange environment for both of us as we were both from families with limited income. The only reason we could afford the sport was that, in an attempt to encourage young talent, membership for juniors where we played was virtually free. To mix with the upper realms of society made us feel like we were something special and we loved it. We were well known at the club for playing whatever the weather. I had even turned up during the snow the previous winter. If I couldn't be a musician, then I hoped to be involved in professional golf in some way. It was my second love.

After our round of golf in the morning, we watched the FA cup final on television in the afternoon. I fell asleep for the entire ninety minutes. It seemed that as my dizziness continued I was becoming more and more exhausted. I stayed the night over at James's house, and although still not feeling right, I continued to fight what was happening in my body. The next day we decided to play golf again.

We started as usual teeing off at the first tee. By this time I was feeling extremely drained and my body was really struggling. However, I had felt tired before at the start of a round of golf, and, once begun, it had always passed. Today was seemingly different though. By the second hole I was far from feeling better. Yet, I decided to push on. It was a beautiful summer day, and I had been playing well recently. I didn't see why I should have to spend my holiday resting.

By the start of the fourth hole I just wanted to sleep. The fourth hole at Betchworth Park, where James and I played, was a long par four where you teed off from an elevated position over 150 yards of heather. James made a great 250-yard drive right down the middle of the fairway. It was my turn. I had just bought a new driver, which I had been dreaming about having for several years. I had finally saved the money and purchased it for myself as a reward for working so hard toward my exams. This was a perfect opportunity to test out my new toy: a long straight hole with the added distance brought by teeing off from an elevated position. I didn't care. By now I just craved sleep like I had not been to bed for days. I managed a feeble drive off to the right hand side, barely clearing the bracken and bunkers.

James knew that I had been feeling under the weather and could see how much I was having to battle with my body to drag myself along the path, through the bracken, towards my ball in the rough.

"Are you sure you wanna keep going?" he asked. "We have all summer to play, why not go home and get some kip?"

"No, I'm alright," I tried to reassure him.

"Well at least take my trolley," James offered.

Although reluctant to make James carry his bag, which was substantially heavier, I really was exhausted.

"If you're sure, that would be cool," I weakly thanked him.

We attached my bag to the trolley and continued towards my ball. After walking another hundred yards, I had to sit down. I just didn't feel I could walk another step.

"Do you mind if we call it a day?" I mumbled.

"Sure, you look like hell," offered a concerned looking James. "There is no way this is a hangover."

"I know," was all I could think of to say, becoming increasingly worried at what might really be wrong with me.

I tried to get up, but stumbled back down again. My legs just didn't seem able to take the weight of the rest of my body. The dizziness of the past days had also reached a new climax. My head felt like it was no longer even attached to my shoulders. I knew things were bad; I just didn't know how bad.

James took my bag, and I eventually managed the short walk back to the clubhouse. I got a lift home and went straight to bed. Lying in that bed should have been the greatest relief of my life. It wasn't. Lying in the bed itself was an effort.

As was often the case during illness, I stayed at my grandparents. It was actually here that I spent much of my childhood. My mother worked full time as a company secretarial assistant, and afterwards in the evening she taught the piano four evenings a week, and then also on Saturday mornings. My stepfather had worked shift work since before he and my mum had married when I was seven. As a consequence, there was rarely anyone available at home between 9:00 in the morning and 7:30 in the evening. My grandmother believed that my sister and I needed more attention than was available at home, and so insisted that we return from school to her and my grandfather's house until our mother had finished teaching. We would then return home for a few hours, where we would sit in front of the television upstairs on our own.

As I spent the next few days sleeping and watching television, no one really gave my health another thought. Everyone assumed that what I was experiencing was due to exam stress and that a good rest would see me back to full health. My grandmother took me to the doctor after a couple of days, just to make sure nothing serious was wrong. I had the usual blood and urine tests, but everything came back as being normal. A virus was decided to be the cause, something the doctor told me it was not possible to test for. The diagnosis seemed logical to me. I had been stressed, and certainly hadn't had as much sleep as I should have. I was informed that such a scenario is classic conditioning to weaken the immune system, and so invite a virus to enter the body.

My energy levels changed very little over the next couple of weeks, although rest did begin to bring more of a relief. Apart from intense fatigue and dizziness, I also developed pains in my muscles and joints. My legs especially troubled me. I had often suffered from aching legs when tired in the past, and this seemed to be the case now more than ever before.

My prime concern was that I still had two exams left. They were both Design and Realisation papers, and together were worth fifty percent of my final mark for that course. For a few days it seemed that it might be impossible for me to take them, as they were two and half hours each and just getting out of bed meant the room would spin uncontrollably. The thought of missing the exams due to illness was hard to take, especially as I had worked so incredibly hard for my coursework.

I had made an electric guitar. The rest of the class had ruthlessly mocked me all year, thinking the idea ridiculously over-ambitious. They had designed and built simple things like model boats or rabbit hutches. The mocking had only made me more determined as I spent many lunchtimes and extra hours after school trying to complete my invention. It had been a true labour of love. Time had ended up getting the better of me, but despite not finishing completely, I had still scored the highest mark in the year. It felt great to succeed against the odds.

Fortunately, by the time the exams came my energy had improved just enough for me to be able to go out of the house for several hours at once. Arrangements were therefore made with the school that I could sit the exams with other students who had special needs, meaning I could leave early if I had to. The day of the first exam came just under two weeks after that first Thursday morning at the hairdressers. I thankfully managed to get through it with few problems.

By the second exam, a couple of days later, I was actually starting to regain significantly more of my energy. In the evening afterwards, Emily and I went to an end of exams party to celebrate our final freedom. Despite still feeling better I ended up only staying a couple of hours. As the evening had gone on, it had become more and more difficult to fit in with my friends without drinking any alcohol. I hadn't touched a drop since the previous party, as the last thing that I wanted was to aggravate how I was feeling. I just hoped that life would get completely back to normal soon so that I could put my mind back to my three loves: music, sport and Emily.

The next few weeks did start to see even more of my energy returning and the dizziness finally beginning to subside. I continued to go out for longer and longer periods and began to resume life as I knew it. Within another couple of weeks, I decided I was well enough to start my two summer jobs. Apart from wanting to get back to normality, I also desperately needed the money to fund my holiday to Shropshire later that summer.

My summer jobs were gardening for one of the senior members at the golf club, and working as an office junior at WS Atkins, an engineering company. The first week was no problem, I got tired, but I only worked four days - two gardening, and two at the office. It was not until the second week that things really started to change once more.

I spent the Tuesday mowing the lawn at my gardening job where I was helping to renovate the garden. I was feeling extremely weak again. The mower was very heavy, and there were several acres to be cut. Making the task even more difficult was the fact that the lawn was on an extremely steep hill. My rapidly draining energy meant that what was a challenging task anyway started to become almost unbearable. I sweated and strained in the hot sun, pushing myself all day long. I simply didn't know how to say "no" and just stop. As far as I was concerned my body should have been able to do whatever I asked of it. It had, after all, always done so up until recently.

By the evening I was horribly exhausted. However, I had arranged to go and see Emily – my reward for a long day's work. We decided to go for a short walk together around the recreation park at the back of where she lived. As we reached the lake, we stopped for a few minutes to throw some bread to the ducks.

After running out, we headed toward the other end of the park where the sports pitches were. I was really trying to be cheerful and good company for Emily, but that wasn't how I felt. I was increasingly frustrated with my health and how it just seemed to be going from bad to worse. I told myself that it was my problem though, trying as much as I could to be the person that I knew she wanted me to be.

The morning after

As we walked past the sports pitches, I spotted someone I knew from some of my classes at secondary school training with the local football team. I tried to watch. Something was not right with my vision. Everything seemed blurred and I just couldn't focus properly. I somehow knew my eyes were fine, yet something clearly wasn't. The more I tried to focus, the more blurred everything became. My heart started to race with anxiety. What the hell was happening to me? Why had I not recovered after a few weeks' rest? What else could I do? How I longed to just run around and forget about the bizarre symptoms I was experiencing. However, I had more pressing things to worry about: tomorrow I was due to work at the office.

It was a gorgeous summer morning as I set off for the train at 8:15. The warming sun reflecting off the car windscreens onto my tanned skin reminded me of how much I normally loved this time of year. Playing sport at every opportunity meant I was always out in the sun developing a great suntan. That was who I was, an active and energetic teenager. The more I was losing touch with that, the more I was losing touch with myself. I was starting to see a different kind of me. I didn't like it.

I arrived at the office in plenty of time and started going about my usual duties of photocopying and typing. The feelings of the previous weeks were back with a vengeance. I was dizzy and tired, and increasingly struggling to concentrate. However, I had already started working three weeks late for the summer due to what was happening to my health, and although I had quite a lot of control over my hours, there was work that people were expecting done. I decided to push on. I hadn't passed out in the hairdressers. Why should I now?

When lunchtime came I went for the usual walk, in the hope that it would ease my feelings of dizziness and exhaustion. It hadn't worked in the past, but it would again give me space. I headed towards the town, listening to my Walkman as I walked. My head was filling with anxiety. What was going on? I had already taken a good few weeks' rest. It was becoming abundantly clear that I did not have a simple virus infection. Why was this happening to me? Suddenly the music on my Walkman became flat and started to slow down. It quickly came to a stop. For a minute I wondered what was happening, but it soon clicked; the batteries had run out. I headed towards the newsagents to get some new ones.

Before I knew it my lunch hour was gone and it was time to return to the office. I had been putting off what I had to do that afternoon for

13

as long as I could. I had to make telephone calls to other companies on the mailing list to update the WS Atkins database. I hated using the telephone, especially to people I didn't know. However, I couldn't say anything to my boss. I had been brought up to please other people over myself, and that is what I attempted to do.

I eventually plucked up the courage to make the first call. It was a wrong number. I tried the next one. The company had moved. The fear was rising; I was feeling worse than I had done in weeks. I tried to fight it, promising myself that after today I would take it easy again. I called the next number on the list. This time I got through and was able to ask the list of questions I had in front of me. The person was helpful, which surprised me. I wasn't used to being treated with kindness. I decided perhaps it mightn't be that bad.

After I finished the call, I got up to go to the toilet. A huge wave of nausea and dizziness swept over me and I dropped back in the chair. I felt horrific. After a few minutes, I managed to stumble to the toilets and sat down in one of the cubicles. Hiding from the world for a while, I attempted to reassess.

As I sat there, trying to understand what was happening, I began to notice how, like the night before, I couldn't focus properly. This was becoming scarily familiar. The room was blurred, but, once again, I knew there was nothing wrong with my eyesight. The problems seemed to be with my balance. What on earth would cause my balance to be affected?

I wanted to wretch my guts out into the toilet and have some visible expression of the horror that I felt inside. Yet, somehow there was no release. I wanted to scream, but again I couldn't; I was too scared to cause a commotion. I just tried to swallow my suffering and push on, hoping that everything would be okay. However, even swallowing normally was starting to feel wrong. My entire body just didn't seem to be working the way it was designed to. My balance, my heart, my eyes, my swallow reflex, they were all going wrong; what was happening to me?

I still had three hours of the working day left. Yet, I was ahead of schedule and so could call it a day if I had to. But I didn't want to go home early. It would mean losing money and could also get me a bad reputation. I questioned inside: why should I have to keep missing out on my summer of freedom? My stubbornness and determination kicked in and I pushed myself to continue. I decided on no more telephone calls though. I just did some simple typing and tried to keep my head low. I thankfully managed to get a couple of naps with my head on the desk when no one was watching. I felt even further sickened by my having to do this just to survive the day.

By the time I got to bed that night, I was as ill as ever. It was quite obvious that something serious was wrong. However, I was an optimist. How bad could it really be? Surely I would get better with time? Thankfully, at that stage I never dwelled on how much time.

CHAPTER 3: WHAT, ME? THE REALITY HITS ME

Peace comes from within.
Do not seek it without.
Buddha

As I sat with my grandmother in the waiting room at my local doctor's practice, I had a looming sense of trepidation at what might be said. It had been two months now since I had first become sick, and it seemed that as time went on I was developing more and more symptoms. The worst thing was that no one seemed to know what they were symptoms of.

I looked at the other patients around me and wondered what was wrong with them. For the three in front of me it seemed fairly obvious. There was a middle-aged man who had his hand in plaster, a young woman who kept sneezing, and a baby who was constantly crying. God, I wished that baby would shut up. What in the past would have been slightly annoying was now giving me a thumping headache. Even my tolerance for noise was becoming severely affected by my deteriorating health.

"How about me?" I wondered. "I look like there is nothing wrong with me; probably none of the other patients could guess why I am here. Yet, I feel like I am close to death much of the time. Patient, what a bloody stupid word," my internal disillusionment continued, "I am more of an impatient." At least I wasn't an inpatient.

I was thankful for one thing: I was out of the house. Even though I would have to sleep for the rest of the day once I got home, at least I would have accomplished something. I had been spending my time the past two months becoming intimately acquainted with the same two pieces of furniture: my bed and the living room sofa. Of course on occasions I did also have the added variety of a voyage to the bathroom.

I had given up hope of an overnight cure, but I was expecting the doctor to have some sort of news today. He had been useless so far. His only idea had been that I had a heart murmur. It had seemed like a logical explanation at the time, for if my body were not getting enough blood, then that would obviously lead to exhaustion and feelings of dizziness. I had almost been hoping that a heart murmur was the source of my problems, for at least then I would have a diagnosis. I was to be disappointed. The specialist that I saw had pointed out that, although I did have a murmur, it was harmless and certainly not the cause of my symptoms.

Upon returning to my GP I had had more blood tests, but, again, they had come back "normal." Yet, I felt very far from "normal." It was taking me time to get used to the idea that no one seemed to know what was wrong with me. I had been brought up to believe that if we get ill, we take a pill, and then we feel better. I had never even considered that there wouldn't be a pill that I could take, let alone being ill and no one having any real idea why. The old "magic formula" of illness + pill = cure, was appearing less and less magical to me.

It had crossed everyone's mind that I might have glandular fever, but again the tests had proved negative. This had been a major relief. The son of one of my grandmother's friends had suffered from glandular fever for over a year now and was still unable even to do a full day at school. I couldn't conceive of many situations worse than being bed bound for such a long period. The last two months had been bad enough. I was an active person with my life revolving around sport and going out. I wondered what you would do with yourself spending a year resting. Life would lose purpose with nothing to do. Luckily I had been cleared. Anyway, such things happened to other people. This was me, my life. I was about action and energy. Sitting around doing nothing wasn't in my character. The word boredom hadn't even been in my vocabulary until recently.

Looking at my grandmother next to me, I could sense that she was also worried. It wasn't often that she was lost for an explanation. This scared me even more. It was days away from my sixteenth birthday, but a part of me still believed that adults knew the answer to most things.

Eventually we were called into the doctor's office. My usual doctor was away on holiday and so for the last few visits I had been seeing one of his partners, Dr. Young. Not that this mattered; they both seemed equally useless. Dr. Young was middle-aged, had short, thinning blonde hair, and a round face and body. I filled him in on the events of the past two weeks. This didn't take long. The only thing to report was that I had developed a couple of additional symptoms: I was getting headaches, and there was a ringing in my ears at night. Dr. Young checked my ears, but could see nothing wrong. This was a response I was getting very used to.

"It must be tinnitus," said Dr. Young. "Not to worry, it will pass. There is nothing I can do about it."

"Well what is wrong with me?" I asked, trying to conceal my frustration.

17

"I'm not really sure," he responded.

"Do you think it could be ME?" my grandmother asked.

I looked round with what must have been a bemused expression on my face.

"I must confess that ME is the most likely explanation," Dr. Young reluctantly replied.

I was too confused to say anything at first. "ME, what is that?" I wondered to myself. The only person I had known with ME was an overweight teacher at my primary school. I had nothing in common with her. There was one thing that I did know about this ME: it was bad news. How bad it was I didn't know.

An uneasy silence descended over the room. It seemed they were waiting for me to say something.

"Well what does that mean?" I managed to ask, still in a state of shock. "Is there a medication I can take or something?"

"No, I'm afraid there is nothing I can give you. You will just have to wait and see what happens," Dr. Young replied.

"Well how long will that take?" I asked, becoming more and more worried, not really prepared for the truth. Thankfully, no one even dared dream the truth back then.

"It's very hard to say," responded Dr. Young. "Sometimes it takes much longer than others. However, I have a good feeling about your case. I think three months should see a world of difference."

Three months, that was a lot worse than I thought. A lot, lot worse. On the other hand, at least I had a diagnosis, I reasoned with myself. And, at least I would be able to play sport again by Christmas.

"I can offer you counselling," Dr. Young solemnly ventured. "We are participating in some research into the effects of counselling in the treatment of ME."

"What do I need counselling for?" I wondered. "I was fit and healthy up until my body gave up on me. There is nothing wrong with my mind. He can't find anything wrong, so he just assumes it's psychological. What an arrogant wanker." Yet, I hid my true feelings and declined politely as I had been brought up to do. However, my grandmother decided she would take the leaflets anyway. By this point I was really biting my tongue. Did she not trust me? Did she believe I was funny in the head as well? Did they think that I was not man enough to cope with this?

Had I had more energy, I would have walked home. However, even the privilege of throwing a normal teenage tantrum was no longer mine. I was dependent on those around me, and that meant doing what I was told or suffering the consequences. As we got into the car, there was only one thought on my mind: "Counselling, how ridiculous. I need medication or something, not some weirdo trying to play with my mind."

A few days later my sixteenth birthday arrived. Because of my fragile state, celebrations amounted to Emily coming around to watch television with me for a couple of hours. This was hardly how I had originally envisioned us spending my sixteenth birthday. I worked very hard to ignore the reality of what my life was rapidly becoming. I knew that things can't have been much fun for Emily either. It wasn't just my summer that was being ruined. I was starting to realise how many of my friends relied on me for enjoying their free time. James was lost with no one to play golf with, the band was hardly rehearsing now, and Emily was spending her time with her cousin sitting around bored. I wasn't the only one who wished things were different.

My birthday also meant making a symbolic telephone call to cancel my summer holiday. It was only two weeks away and there was no way that I would be well enough to go. I was supposed to be joining a group of friends that I had met on holiday in Shropshire the year before for a week of outdoor activities. What was meant to be the icing on top of my summer of dreams was also being stolen from me. How did I feel? I continued to try not to. I just gritted my teeth and got on with life.

My contact with the outside world was rapidly becoming more and more distant. An average week amounted to long periods of sleep, interspersed with television and a couple of visits and telephone calls from Emily. It never dawned on my friends that they could have just come and sat with me for an hour or two. Perhaps the fact that I didn't even care was a testament to how much my priorities and state of mind had changed. Even being with Emily was meaning less to me. I liked the idea of having a girlfriend, yet I just didn't have any passion left inside me. I was far too concerned with getting enough energy just to be able to go out of the house for more than a doctor's visit. Emily and I were slowly drifting apart and, like the rest of my life, I felt like there was nothing I could do about it.

GCSE's results also came and went. Just collecting them was difficult. I had to sleep in the car for the short journey to school, and then go through the torment of trying to look happy and like nothing was wrong with me. My friends knew I was ill, but the last thing I wanted was to appear weak. I had had too many experiences of bullying to risk ridicule.

My results were, by most peoples' standards, excellent. By my family's standards, they were quite poor. I got three A's, five B's and one C. I didn't really care anyway. I knew I could have done better if I had chosen to. Studying wasn't where my priorities lay. I had given up trying to be an academic achiever years ago. What I did had never been good enough for those around me. Soon the academic pressure would start again. I could hardly wait.

CHAPTER 4: A NEW START? (AUTUMN 1996 AND PRE-1996)

The most spiritual human beings, assuming they are the most
courageous, also experience by far the most painful tragedies; but
it is precisely for this reason that they honour life, because it brings
against them its most formidable weapons.
Friedrich Nietzsche

As I lay on my bed at my grandparents listening to the radio, on came "Oh Yeah," by Ash. It was a song that I had been listening to constantly while revising for my GCSE's, back before I became ill. As I listened to the opening words my mind drifted back three months; back to when my life had been full of hope and dreams. Since then the summer had passed and I had done almost nothing apart from sleep, watch television, and witness my life disappearing around me. I guess there was one benefit to my new lifestyle: I could win any debate on the reasons why Anne Wilkinson was the best-looking character in "Neighbours," my favourite television show. Some people make a great social life out of such knowledge, but for me it was just another cruel reminder of how pathetic my life had become.

On the positive side, my energy had slowly started to improve. In the last few weeks I had actually been able to go out of the house for several hours at a time. As long as I restrained from physical activity and took regular rests, I could also stay awake for most of the day. Tomorrow I was starting at a new school for sixth form and, with my health possibly returning, I was beginning to get excited about a potential fresh start, a new me. I prayed that I might finally be able to leave the past behind. It had been pretty horrific.

My older sister by two years, Georgina (George), had become anorexic when I was eleven years old. She was so ill at one stage that her weight had dropped below six and a half stones and she was staring death in the face. It was only through a top London clinic that some weight was forced back on her. Her illness created an ongoing war-zone at home. At times she was violent, others abusive, and living with her was always like being in the presence of a ticking time bomb.

I remember one time when George ran away from the clinic and was trying to evade going back. With the police and family searching for her, she had been found, and had just stopped off at our grandparents to collect a few things before returning to the clinic. She was begging not to be made to go back, and so escape being forced to regain a healthy body weight. Without the clinic she would almost certainly die, as her body was already so desperate for food that it was digesting her muscles. Mum was crying and begging George to go back peacefully, having already been bruised severely in attacks from her earlier in the day. With Mum's ageing parents there, the situation was terrifyingly volatile.

At this moment George was not the sister that had I grown up with. It was like she was possessed. I could barely look her in the eyes. They were terrifying, like the devil in some badly made horror film: bloodshot and swollen with anger and hate. She was both scared out of her mind and totally enraged at the same time.

We were all in the dining room. The connecting bathroom door had just been broken down to get George out. She had locked herself in there over an hour ago threatening to kill herself.

"I'm not going back, you can't make me," she screamed at our distraught mother threateningly.

"You have no choice, without it you will die," Mum pleaded, attempting to block George's path to the front door, desperate to make her see sense.

"No, I hate that place, I'm so fat. You don't understand, no one understands me," George shrieked.

"George, I love you, you know that. That is why you must return, it breaks my heart to see you like this," begged Mum.

"Fuck you. I hate you. I hate you all. You all want me dead anyway," George savagely attacked.

I was eleven years old and watching all the people close to me tearing each other apart. I felt totally helpless and totally alone. Those that I looked up to in life, those I should have been able to turn to for guidance and support, were all in absolute despair. The situation was totally unpredictable and completely out of control. No one knew what to do. Getting the police further involved would be risky; in this state George could end up being violent towards them and so add a criminal record to her already immense problems.

Suddenly George made a lunge for Mum, punching her, kicking her and attacking her in any way possible. Mum was desperately trying to defend herself, while also trying to restrain George. It wasn't working. George was desperate and ruthless. She pulled off Mum's glasses and smashed them on the floor, before striking her again in the face several more times. She was going to do whatever it took to break free. But what would she be breaking free to? If she were not killed living on the streets, then she would probably starve herself to death. There was no way she could be allowed to escape. Someone had to do something and fast.

I was nearest, and probably the only person in the room who was stronger than George. I hated violence, but I was going to have to choose to act, or live with the consequences of doing nothing. If I did nothing, my mother could be severely hurt and George even die. But, if I did do something, I could injure my own sister. I was lost. I wanted more than anything for the whole thing just to end. Such thoughts were secondary though, as so often seemed the case when I was a child, I had to ignore my own needs. The survival of my family was in my hands.

I grabbed George by her long brunette hair and pulled her to the ground. She tried to fight me off, but there was little she could do. I had a firm grip, and under her maniac exterior she was still only six and half stone, not much against my at the time overweight ten stone. "Stop it, you're hurting me!" George screamed, frothing at the mouth like an animal.

"Calm down," I begged. "Stop struggling, please." My heart was aching for what I was being forced to do. My pain was only numbed by the urgency of the situation.

After a while George lay still, admitting temporary defeat. However, it was not over. She still had to return to the clinic. What would face her then? More battles with those around her, those that deep down she loved? More struggles to just perform one of life's most simple actions, eating food? In that moment life felt so futile. What could anyone do?

Eventually George had to be carried kicking and screaming into the car, before being driven back to the clinic, with the help of my stepfather who had subsequently arrived. This was after she decided to have one final go at escape and had destroyed the few antiques in our grandparent's hall that had escaped her aggression on previous days. My memories of my sister from the age of ten onwards are filled with similar scenes.

Although the staff at the clinic did force some weight back on George, they also gave her a whole set of new problems. They essentially achieved weight gain using a diet consisting of masses of chocolate, crisps and junk food and, when necessary, force-feeding. My sister went into the clinic with an eating disorder and she came out with the seeds of mental illness.

Within a very short period of George being discharged from the clinic the situation at home was so bad that she was put into foster care. I have quite a poor memory of much of this period and to be honest I am glad. From what I do remember, my mum and stepfather nearly divorced as the nightmare of my sister's situation spread. I also know that I often lived in fear of what was going to happen next. Sometimes I would break down crying at school, but soon the only way I could find to survive was by bottling my emotions up. I learnt that if no one else cared about how I was coping, I mustn't be worth worrying about.

As anorexia nervosa became less of a problem, George developed anorexia bulimia. This meant that she was eating vast quantities of food and then purging, either by deliberately making herself sick, taking vast quantities of laxatives, or exercising excessively. It isn't difficult to guess the influence that the feeding regimes used at the original anorexia clinic had had on George's new eating behaviours. The situation soon, once again, became so extreme that she was in serious danger of dying, this time from liver and intestinal damage.

Many attempts were made to stop George's self-destructive behaviours, such as locking food in the garage at home to limit her eating, and placing her photograph behind the desk of every chemist in our local area to prevent her from buying laxatives. However, nothing seemed to work long-term; George was always intelligent enough to find a way around. The same genius she used to excel academically, and in sport and music, she was also using to destroy herself.

By her late teens, George's anorexia bulimia did fade into the background. The new label was depression, with her even being sectioned under the Mental Health Act, deemed too dangerous to herself and others to be left alone. By this time her suicide attempts had also became more and more extreme, and where interspersed with bouts of serious self-harming, such as using razor blades to cut her arms and legs until there was barely an inch of skin untouched. Soon all the knives and sharp objects in the house had to also be locked up with the food. There only seemed to be one solution: to try and survive from day to day and hope that things got better.

By the time George was twenty, her depression and suicidal tendencies had developed into severe violence towards family members, accompanied by manic-depression (also known as bipolar disorder). Of the dozens of psychiatrists and psychologists that were involved, there was not a single one that made a positive difference. She simply told them lies, along with the police, about how she had been abused and horrifically treated by various family members. Sometimes she was believed, meaning various family members ended up in the local police station. The rest of the time the authorities, like the rest of us, had no idea what to do.

George's battles to find a satisfying and fulfilling life were an endless cause of pain for those closest to her. There were many times when I was growing up that I hated her, feared her, and was jealous of the attention she gained. At really desperate times, I even wished that she would actually kill herself as she so often tried to, ending the pain for everyone who was being hurt by her.

Whilst these events with my sister were happening, my relationships with others close to me were equally horrendous. My grandmother and I battled every day over my schoolwork. My aspirations to be a musician were a constant bone of contention, with band practice having soon been limited to once a week. My grandmother thought it was the right thing. I didn't agree. We both wanted me to be successful; we just had different ideas as to what success meant. The fact that I was top of the class in almost all of my subjects was simply not enough to earn me the right to live my dreams. I was told that music was for the "low life," and I was not to mix with them. Being determined as I was, arguments were constant.

It seemed that the more George fell out of line, the more it was decided that I had to make up for it. By the time I was at secondary school George was hardly around at home, spending most of her time either in foster care, in a mental hospital, or at boarding school. I would therefore be at my grandparents alone for about four hours after school, until my grandmother drove me home for when Mum finished teaching the piano at around 7:30, ready to let her know that I had been "misbehaving" again. I used to dread it so much. I didn't see Mum very often, and because of these daily episodes with my grandmother most of the time we spent together was contaminated by having to repair the "damage" of my apparent "misbehaviour."

I found it incredibly hard to comprehend why I was being treated the way I was. Did my family not understand that I was doing well enough at school and that I was only learning to hate studying by being forced to do extra work at home, I would continually question. My only reward was when I earned a bit of praise, but it seemed that I had to be top of the class by a considerable margin to win this. After every mark it was not, "Congratulations, I am so proud of you!" It was more like, "Where was that compared to everyone else?" If I was not top, then came the inevitable question, "Well who was top then?" I could feel the disappointment in the air, and there was then the usual, said more to themselves than anyone else, "You'll do better next time."

Once mum had been told of my terrible behaviour at my grandmother's, and how I was not welcome there again, the guilt trip set in. Did I not appreciate everything that my grandparents did for me? Where would I go to after school if I were not welcome there? Did I think that Mum was made of money and that she could afford a childminder (although it did come to that once)? Next came the dreaded question: what was I going to do to make things right? By this stage I was often even starting to believe that I was in the wrong. After all, everyone else seemed so sure. What was the opinion of a misunderstood child worth?

Once my lecture on how to be perfect was over, it was time for me to apologise. I always agreed to do so. I just couldn't bear the thought of adding to the already immense suffering of those around me. I would swallow my pride, and my own sense of self with it, and telephone my grandmother to tell her that I was sorry I was so ungrateful and unloving, and that I hurt her so much. Ultimately, I was sorry for being me. Often I would also add an excuse to help in the process, anything to take some of the overwhelming feeling of blame off my shoulders. Each night I was eventually forgiven and told that I was welcome back the next day. Every so often my grandmother was even sorry that she had shouted too, but that was saved for special occasions. That one needed a real bust up.

My family situation was the way it was, in part, because my mother and real father divorced soon after I was born. A few months after that, he was seen for the last time. I knew very little about him, only his name, that he had a beard, and a few minor details about his life. I actually spent very little of my childhood thinking of him. I guess it is hard to miss something you never had.

My mother remarried when I was seven. My stepfather and I were never close. For a time I hoped we might be, but the constant battles in our home, much contributed to by my sister's increasing troubles and my grandmother's dominance, seemed to just push him away. On several occasions our home was put on the market as my mother prepared to divorce him, yet it never actually went through. I have to say, in defence of my stepfather, I am not sure I would have stuck around considering how horrific things often got. He had a choice and I didn't. He may have been a lousy stepfather, but at least he didn't abandon us.

CHAPTER 5: SOMEONE HELP ME PLEASE

A man who suffers much, knows much; every day brings him
new wisdom.
Ewe

It became abundantly clear that I needed some form of treatment, but from where? I had little idea where to start. The doctor's offer of counselling had turned out to be a joke, except no one was laughing. My mum and grandmother had coerced me into going, but I knew I should have stuck with my instincts. I had been asked pointless questions about my past and offered useless advice from someone who was living in another generation. I am sure that the counsellor had meant well, but there was about an ice cube's chance in hell of it benefiting me. I simply couldn't see how spending my time focusing on all the bad things in my life was going to make me feel any better. After all, I'd never heard of anyone finding health or happiness searching through rubbish. As far as I was concerned it would just be a great way to create more depression and hopelessness. I decided I already had enough of that in my life and so I quit after two sessions.

With the failure of the counselling, my doctor's only offer of help, it became apparent that traditional treatment had nothing left to offer me, and it was at this point that I turned my back on it and looked to the alternative/complementary therapies instead. It seemed I was in luck. A friend of my grandmother's was a practitioner of the Bowen technique and was able to give me an appointment almost immediately.

The Bowen technique is a therapy that works on the idea that illness is caused by blocked energy. With the skilful manipulation of various energy points around the body, this energy can be freed up and so either directly or indirectly assist in healing. In the leaflet I was given at my first visit, there was the case study of a girl around my age who had been totally cured of ME in only a few sessions. This sounded pretty good! If it could be done for her, then why not for me, I convinced myself, reasoning that I must be in the right place now.

Three months later I was less optimistic. There had not been a single change, despite weekly appointments; I had simply spent another ten weeks of my life in bed, sleeping, watching television, and struggling to do a couple of hours school a day. Although I was told that I would still benefit from occasional treatments, it was clear to everyone that the answers for me did not lie here. I wondered to myself about the girl in the leaflet. Her ME had totally disappeared almost overnight. Why was the same not happening for me? Why was I any different? In fact, why was this happening to me at all? What had I done to deserve ME? Why me? Surely I had already had enough suffering in my life? Such questions might have been useless, but I was still asking them.

In her continued quest to help me recover, my grandmother had been researching possible treatment plans for ME. Through her reading she had discovered some potentially helpful vitamins and herbal remedies, which I had been taking. She had also come across the idea that ME can be caused by an overgrowth of candida albicans, a form of mould that resides primarily in our digestive systems. The books that she had been reading listed some of the symptoms of a candida overgrowth as extreme fatigue, dizziness, headaches and muscle pains. I was pretty stunned; these were exactly my symptoms!

The books explained that a candida overgrowth can occur in a number of ways: through a high sugar diet, severe stress, and also by taking many of modern medicines "magic pills," especially antibiotics, steroids and the contraceptive pill. It seemed that I fulfilled most of these criteria. Although not untypical, my diet was hardly healthy; I was quite partial to chocolate, crisps, and sweets, as well as having an insatiable appetite for coca-cola. As a child I had also had significant amounts of antibiotics and had clearly been no stranger to stress. The important question was; had my lifestyle been bad enough to cause a candida overgrowth? Because there seemed to be no accurate way of testing, and also because traditional doctors did not recognise candida as a cause of ME, there was no real way of knowing apart from giving the treatment a try.

According to my grandmother's research, there were four aspects of treatment necessary to deal with a candida overgrowth. Firstly, to kill the candida using anti-fungal drugs; secondly, to replenish the supply of "good" bacteria in the digestive system with probiotics. Thirdly, to support the immune system using nutritional supplements and, finally, to stop feeding the candida by removing certain foods from the diet. The last part was initially rather a shock, for foods that feed candida include sugar, fruit, yeast, alcohol and coffee. This basically meant saying goodbye to puddings and snacks as I knew them, and therefore also leaving behind one of the few pleasures I had left in life. But, in a strange kind of way, I actually didn't mind, really for one simple reason: I finally felt like I had something that I could actively do to help myself.

28

Once again though, having been on the programme for several months, the benefits were distinctly lacking. Thankfully, my grandmother continued her research, and in doing so she came across a local doctor, Dr. Mansfield, who specialised in the treatment of candida. An appointment was made, and I must confess that I was relieved to once again have some professional assistance.

It was a cold and wet November morning when my grandmother accompanied me for my first visit. Dr. Mansfield's practice was set in a large house, which also accommodated an osteopath and an allergy centre. The waiting room was in the hall and offered encouraging first impressions. Browsing through several of Dr. Mansfield's books - on allergies, arthritis, and general diet control, the seemingly countless case studies of patients experiencing dramatic healing gave my belief in Dr. Mansfield a boost. I just hoped that this was not going to be a repeat of my reading about recovery being as far as things went.

After sitting for a while, a middle-aged man with side parted brown hair and a good physique jogged down the staircase in front of us, introduced himself as Dr. Mansfield, and welcomed us up to his office on the first floor. As I struggled to drag my weak body up the stairs, I quietly said a prayer to myself, "Please God, let this be it. I will do whatever it takes to be healthy, please just give me my life back." I sincerely hoped someone was listening.

Once inside the office, we sat down and Dr. Mansfield started questioning me on the minute details of my medical history. He explained that he was not only interested in my recent problems, but also everything I had experienced in the past with regard to both my physical and psychological well-being. To me this was novel. I had never met a doctor before who was concerned with more than just my symptoms.

When I was very young I had had fluid on my eardrums and T-tubes had been fitted to assist drainage. The T-tube in my right ear had in time slipped and left a hole, resulting in two skin graft operations to repair the damage. Despite appearing totally irrelevant, this had been of considerable interest (I eventually discovered that the original fluid was probably due to a milk intolerance), as was the fact I had had adult size tonsils at the age of five, which were subsequently removed. Especially of pertinence were the stomach problems I had experienced throughout most of my teens.

From about the age of thirteen I had regularly suffered with what had eventually been diagnosed as Irritable Bowel Syndrome (IBS).

This essentially meant that on an almost daily basis I had to excuse myself from class to go and sit in agony on the toilet until I could force a bowel movement. Often the pain was so intense that there seemed to be nothing I could do but sit as still as possible, force myself to breathe and wait for it to pass. Over recent months my IBS had become less and less of a problem and I had started to forget about those countless mornings of agony. That was up until now. Suddenly my IBS was very relevant. According to Dr. Mansfield, it was an obvious example of dietary problems, as he believed my ME to also be. The fact that the pains had recently reduced as I had changed my diet seemed to suggest he was correct.

It suddenly struck me how obvious the role of diet in IBS is. Our stomach's function is to digest food; consequently, just like if you put diesel into an unleaded car it is going to ruin the engine, any problems with our stomachs are most likely to be because they are struggling to handle what we are eating. This was hardly a complicated idea! Why the hell then had the stomach specialist I had visited three years previously not even inquired in passing about my diet? As I sat there in front of Dr. Mansfield, it seemed almost criminal to me how the medical profession had failed me.

I was just beginning to understand the massive shortcomings of modern medicine, its almost total failure with many of society's most prevalent illnesses. I developed this theory that you could go along to many doctors suffering from something as simple as headaches and be given pills to remove them. But, because your body doesn't like the pills it would raise your blood pressure in response. No doubt the doctor would have something for this too, but this might then give you constipation. However, never fear, the chances are there would be something for this also. Before you knew it, on a daily basis you would be taking ten different pills, and experiencing a whole bunch of side effects – symptoms that weren't even there before. And then, lo and behold, twenty years later you could have a heart attack, caused by, you guessed it: stress. Incredibly, your doctor would have managed to stop your body's warning that your lifestyle needed adjusting, otherwise known as a headache, twenty years ago!

However, this was not meant as an attack on doctors; I was aware that many of them go into the profession with the aim of helping people. Medical school is an incredibly challenging place where in a short space of time students are forced to remember massive amounts of information, with almost no opportunity to question what they are

30

being taught. Before they know it our doctors have studied for over seven years and seen very little back for their efforts. The last thing they are going to want to do is discard what they have been intensely learning, in search of something that, although potentially more effective, goes against everything they have been indoctrinated in.

Of course we do not help, for most of us go along wanting a quick fix and to have our symptoms taken away, be this with a pill or something more invasive. However, although there was clearly much justification for the state of Western medicine, at the time it wasn't enough to pacify my growing frustration. I reasoned that surely I had deserved at least access to information with regard to food and diet which, had I followed, may have totally changed my life. As I was starting to learn, it perhaps may even have avoided the mess I was now finding myself in.

I also started to question the example being set by those that are in positions of influence in our society. All the people around me, including my doctors, teachers and family, were all following the same typical high sugar Western diet. How was I to have known that such a lifestyle was dangerous? Sure, healthy living was spoken of, but no one close to me really lived it. Not until they were very desperate, anyway, it seemed.

As my appointment with Dr. Mansfield continued, he explained that there were several possible causes of my present situation. This was exactly what I wanted to hear! Up until this point I had been told that all I could do was rest. Apparently, the easiest contender to analyse first was food intolerances. Dr. Mansfield explained that food intolerances are caused by peoples' bodies having learnt to respond unfavourably to particular foods. If these foods are eaten, the result can be a number of negative symptoms, such as fatigue, dizziness, muscle pains, headaches and tinnitus. Again, these symptoms sounded rather familiar.

The best way to effectively test for any food intolerances that I might have developed, from the perspective of Dr. Mansfield, was to go ten days with eating nothing but totally neutral foods, and then, once my body had de-toxed, to introduce a new food at each meal and monitor the effect. In essence, this meant that for ten days I was to eat nothing but basmati rice, plain fish, lamb, sweet potatoes, carrots and green beans.

I had never been particularly partial to any of the foods on my new menu. As a child I had always been very fussy about food and would

31

eat only two vegetables: peas and potatoes. I had been so adamant that I would touch nothing else, that I had actually become quite skilled at hiding food in my serviette. I figured that if I didn't want to starve, this was going to have to change. As I was to discover, it is amazing how easy it is to transform lifelong patterns of behaviour when we have a compelling enough reason. Knowing that recovering my health might depend upon it, almost over night years of hatred of healthy food disappeared. It was quite a shock to everyone, including me.

As I implemented Dr. Mansfield's regime and waited for the expected results, I tried to keep my head above water at school. My ME symptoms were all the worse for having the added stress. I would come home after a couple of hours in the morning and go straight to bed, resurface about lunch time, have lunch, and then return to bed until the late afternoon. Everything that involved movement of any kind was stressful, and often painful. Walking especially was exhausting, and was also frightening because of the inherent risk of collapsing.

Being with people was becoming harder and harder. I could no longer relate to the world in the same way I had in the past. My current reality was just too alien. What do you say to people about your life when all you do is sleep and watch television? People at St. John's had never known me when I was healthy, and it seemed to me that there was only so much that I could talk about the lives of soap opera characters without sounding like I was a pathetic loser with no life. That was, after all, what I felt I was fast becoming. I therefore learnt to hide as much of my illness from them as I could. Yet, in doing so, I was also hiding my life.

It didn't help that my friends from my last school never visited. They knew that I was ill, but with our friendships having been built around activity, they no longer saw any point in spending time with me. I soon forgot about them as well. It seemed easier just to retreat into my mind and try to escape the nightmare of my life. Falling asleep should have been a great way of doing so. It wasn't. My sleep was also plagued by nightmares. Like the merging of two colours, it was hard to tell where one nightmare ended and the next started. It was also hard to decide which was worse: real life, or my dreams. Both were frightening. I guess at least with a sleeping nightmare you wake up. I couldn't say the same for my waking life. There was never any break and I could see no end in sight, just an uncertain future of illness and despair. All that was left to listen to was my mind and its increasing state of panic and depression. I was becoming more and more terrified, and more and more lost. I was very thankful that someone thought that they had the answer.

It was also around this time that Emily dumped me. We had been at different schools since September, and considering I had seen her only twice in the last two months, our break up was hardly surprising. She called me one day and reeled off the usual spiel, "I think that we'll always be great friends, but we're just not good as a couple anymore." When I came off the telephone I expected to feel hurt, but I wasn't. I was just relieved I would no longer have to worry about her. I knew she deserved better than the measly few minutes on the telephone each night that I could offer. It was bad enough that I was going through hell, why should she have to come with me? At the same time, another chapter of my past had closed. There was very little of life as I had known it remaining. The only pleasure left in my life was a few fried sweet potatoes before bed each night. Hardly the vision I had held for my teenage years.

CHAPTER 6: A NIGHT OF TERROR (WINTER 1996)

That little bit of sadness when you wake up in the morning that you spoke of, I think I know what that is; perhaps you are not doing what you are meant to be doing.
Unbreakable

I tried to focus on the numbers. The telephone was surely such a simple device? I had used it so many times before. But it felt so claustrophobic. Still, there was no time for fear; I had to get through. It was a matter of life or death. I dialled the number, but half way in I knew I had made a mistake. I tried again, just remembering to press the coin return. I only had one coin left; I had already lost so many. I made a tenth and final attempt. Was it ten? How long had I been here? Was I really here? I knew I was me, yet I felt so fearful, so disconnected.

The world around me was feeling more and more hostile. However, before I had time to panic, the fear grabbed me again, like the arm of a giant sweeping me up in its powerful embrace. There was no escape. I had to get through. I dialled one more time. I was nearly there; just a couple more numbers. Ah, oh no, again, I had failed again.

Was there anyone there, someone who could help me? People were just going about their business, completely oblivious to my fear and the urgency of the situation. I tried to look normal and like there was nothing wrong, afraid to cause a commotion. But did no one understand? Surely they could see the danger as well? I began to shake, unable to stand still. I was sweating profusely. My heart was pumping like a machine gun, relentless, no break. "Thump, thump, thump." Empty shells were falling to the ground in the form of sweat. Was I at war? If so, with whom? I had to get through. The world was spinning, I couldn't see properly. Sweat was blocking my eyes; how could I fight if I could not see? "HELP," I tried to scream, but the words became lost in my throat. The panic took over and I began to lose it. The world peeled away. The dark night became total blackness in a matter of seconds.

I jolted up in bed, dripping in sweat and shaking with fear, almost the same as in my nightmare, but the urgency had gone; my surroundings were known once again. I was still alive. Not that it made much difference. I rolled over and tried to get back to sleep, desperately wanting to leave behind the horror that had become my body. My ears were ringing louder than ever. A barely audible monotone had become an overweight opera singer who could only sing one note.

Despite having a thick duvet and pyjamas on, I was still freezing. It seemed the cold world could penetrate anything. Yet it felt like the cold was also on the inside, at the centre of my being. I wondered, what would cause such an experience? I turned in the bed again and tried to curl up into the foetal position, but with my aching legs even that hurt. Shutting my eyes even tighter, I craved for my sleepiness to take me away.

After what seemed like several more hours I looked at my alarm clock, it was only 2:30. I still had six more hours alone in this bed of fear. I just wanted someone to hold me, someone to take away my pain and tell me I was going to make it through. I was too old for that though. I should be stronger than this, I told myself. If I had not been so frightened that if I stood up I would pass out, I might have acted like the scared child I felt and gone to my grandparents' room for some comfort. That was out of the question though. It would mean leaving my fortress and entering the unknown. There may be mutiny inside, but it was surely less scary than what lay outside in the trials and tribulations of that dark corridor.

Ten days after my initial consultation I returned to see Dr. Mansfield. Watching him jog up the stairs as he welcomed us into his office, I was once again reassured. If he had created such vibrant health for himself, then why not in me? He outlined that for the next step of the programme I was to introduce a new food each meal and monitor my body's response. Foods that led to no effect were to be reintroduced into my diet. Any foods that I felt had led to a change in symptoms were to be avoided for the time being, and sugar, wheat, yeast, preservatives, flavourings and additives were not to be eaten for the foreseeable future.

A few weeks later I was back with Dr. Mansfield for a third consultation, disappointed that I was still reaping no benefits. I had felt worse after eating eggs and a few other things, but because I felt terrible the whole time anyway it was very difficult to decipher whether the foods were the actual cause. It seemed to be more life itself that was the source of my symptoms. The next step of my treatment was to begin a full-on assault against candida, which, in the absence of food intolerances, Dr. Mansfield believed to be at the root of my problems.

Dr. Mansfield's anti-candida treatment essentially involved continuing with the sugar and yeast free diet that I was on, with the addition of no fructose (meaning no fruit apart from melon). I was also to start taking Nystatin, a powerful anti-candida drug, to which I was to slowly build up my tolerance. Within a month I was on the full dosage with still no apparent change. Extra tests arranged by Dr. Mansfield had also shown up various mineral deficiencies, and I was consequently given the appropriate supplements. Again, I appeared not to be responding.

As I continued to wait for the programme to take effect, life went on. I say life, it wasn't really a life; my existence still consisted of two main things: sleeping, and struggling to keep up with a few hours school each day. The biggest excitement of my week was going home on a Saturday night to watch a video with my mum and stepfather. If I were feeling up to it in the afternoon, Mum would also take me to the shops for a few minutes after my afternoon rest. However, this was often quite traumatic. Walking any more than a few hundred yards was disastrous and would usually see me completely wiped out. Sometimes the adverse effects would last for days.

Somehow, I had so far managed to keep up with three A-levels; meaning that in theory I should have been attending fourteen or fifteen hours of classes a week. Just sitting through what of these I could was hard, almost unbearably hard. Homework was the worst. For my two hours at school I ran on adrenaline. However, when I returned home, the false mask that I had worn fell to the floor and my reality hit me again. It was hurting more and more. Adding to my pain was the knowing that I was missing out on my teenage years, what were meant to be some of the best years of my life. Many days I didn't even have enough strength to strum the strings on my guitar for a few minutes, let alone contemplate any kind of a social life.

I wish I could say that I cried for what I had lost and what I was missing out on, but I didn't. Maybe it hurt too much? Maybe I was used to life kicking me? I figured that I just had to get on with it, keep my head down and do the best I could. What other choice did I have? I had nowhere else to go. Even if I did, I didn't even have the strength to get there. I had to stay and fight. But with what, and against whom? I wished I knew.

As the monotonous months of illness merged together, January eventually arrived. With it came a place in the category of the chronically ill, for I had now been suffering from ME for over six months. This was another label I could do without. So much for Dr. Young's guess of three months seeing the world of difference. I did

36

not feel an ounce better than I had done at the start. I guess there was one thing for sure; I was finally becoming used to my illness. Yet, with this came a very dangerous shift in my mental health. At the time, it was just my daily experience, and the word "depression" did not exist for me. However, this is exactly what started to happen; I started to fall into a very deep clinical depression. I doubt anyone around me was really aware of my developing despair and disillusionment with life. As I had always done, I acted cheerfully and tried to look like I was coping. The reality was that I wasn't. The world was making less and less sense to me.

Worst of all, depression wasn't just inside me; it was all around. My family members were still using either anti-depressants or alcohol to numb their pain. When I did go to school, I would painfully struggle, sometimes desperately, for a couple of hours before dragging myself to the school gate where my grandmother would meet me to drive me home to bed. That was the only contact that I had with the world. This depression that started to engulf me was something that intensified over the coming months. It was a change in perception that was to take me so low that some things in my life could never be the same again. Still, I had a long way to fall yet.

CHAPTER 7: PLEASE NO MORE, SOMEONE STOP THIS
(WINTER 1996 TO SUMMER 1997)

Nothing happens to any man that he is not formed by nature to bear.
Marcus Aurelius

With the new school term beginning, trying to survive went from a horrible nightmare to the impossible. The intensity of work was growing and I just couldn't keep up. I was becoming severely stressed, and this was just making me even sicker, if that was possible. It didn't help that I had no understanding from my teachers. As far as they were concerned, I was just another pupil who didn't really care about learning. They had never known me when I was healthy, and so assumed that this was who I was, a malingering teenager. They knew that I was ill, but the way they saw it I was just tired. We all get a bit tired sometimes, I would be told.

My life reached a dead-end one Friday night in February. I could take no more. No longer was I able to hold up the immense weight that was continually crushing down on my already weak shoulders. It was a cold and wet evening, and I was feeling my now usual exhausted, spaced out and aching self. I had homework due in the next day and I was seriously struggling to sit at my desk for twenty minutes to get my dizzy head around it.

The driving rain attacking the window in front of me reminded me of life's constant barrages. Would they ever end? All I wanted was to go to sleep, although I was all too aware that I would still have to wake up and face life again. There just seemed to be no way out. In an attempt to lift my mood, I decided to take a couple of minutes away from my dreaded books and I picked up my acoustic guitar. As I sat there attempting to play a few chords and escape the world, it only added to my hopelessness. Something that had used to be the centre of my life had become just another cruel reminder of the life that I now lived. At least on this night I was just about able to strum the strings, I tried to reassure myself. Thank God for small mercies.

Unfortunately, I was not the only one that knew I had homework to complete. My grandmother was still playing her self-appointed role of home tutor. Over recent months she had been fairly tolerant of the fact that I was falling behind, but this was about to change. She knew that I felt like hell, but for her, study was the essence of life, and although my health was in jeopardy, she believed that I should be willing to risk that extra bit of effort. She, like my teachers, couldn't see what was in front of her own eyes. As she passed my room and heard the sound of me playing my guitar, she burst in with a look of horror on her face. "Why are you not doing your work?" she angrily interrogated me. "If you fall any further behind you will have to drop out. You know that without your A-levels you cannot go to university, and then you will have no degree. Where will that leave you? You seem to be perfectly capable of playing that guitar, so why not studying? It is far more important. I've told you before, you will never make a living through music."

It sounded like the same argument that we had had a thousand times. However, this time it was different. Playing the guitar these days wasn't about music stardom; it was about a few minutes escape from my living hell. Did my grandmother not understand that every ounce of energy that I had found that week had been dedicated to trying not to fall behind at school? Did she not understand that this was the first time in days that I had even been able to play my guitar? I decided on avoidance tactics. I was too exhausted to argue. I just wanted to be left alone. My life was bad enough already, could no one see that?

"Do you not care about your future?" she struck again. "You have so much potential, it is terrible to see you waste it like this." Did she think that I did not realise? Was it not obvious that I hated my life? "I don't care," I whimpered in response, desperate to avoid an argument. I was past even being angry; that would take too much energy, energy that I would need to crawl into bed.

Yet, as I sat there trying to ignore my grandmother and her words, my mind started to remind me of what was happening to me: how my life had been stolen for no apparent reason, how I had lost my friends and freedom, not to mention my daily struggles with my health. And how could I ever forget the daily pain, both physical and mental; my endless days alone, with nothing to do but sleep, even when I knew it would make no difference to my exhaustion and never ending muscle aches? The more my reality hit me, the more I could feel the emotion building inside me. Getting to bed was clearly going to have to wait. I was not going to be allowed to retreat. At that moment I couldn't conceive of things becoming any worse. I couldn't hide from the truth anymore.

Before my grandmother could launch her next tactical assault, I felt a mutiny inside. My defences came crashing down. The armour that was defending me from the outside world and keeping my pain inside split open. Out burst an onslaught of emotion.

"I can't do this anymore! I can't do this anymore!" I screamed.

Tears exploded from my eyes, like ammunition in a catapult that had been held back for months. I broke down and collapsed on the bed, shaking with the intensity of the emotion that was being released from within me.

"I can't do this anymore!" I cried continually. "I can't do this anymore!" like a mantra, again and again, I relentlessly shrieked the same words. They seemed to be the only words in my vocabulary, the only words that could express how I felt.

There was nothing left I could do but just feel the pain. My grandmother, taken aback by the effect of her poorly chosen tactics, put her arms around me and held me as I returned my locked up emotion to the universe. There was nothing she could say. I had to let it out. At that moment I was inconsolable; it was a matter of waiting for the waves to become ripples once again. Even she did not feel strong enough to change the flow of a tidal wave.

The pain continued to cleanse me for what seemed liked hours, but after a number of final desperate assaults, the barrage retreated, leaving me further drained, but also strangely peaceful. Months of frustration seemed to have been dissipated for a while. However, even this release did not last long. After a few minutes, the harsh reality of my situation began to strike me all over again. Some of my emotional energy may have been released, but I was still in a desperate place.

There was one thing for sure: there was no way I was continuing with my life the way it was. It had become too much. As my grandmother continued to hold me in her arms, she knew that pushing me would work no longer. It would only lead to less time at school and therefore less of a chance of me living the life she wanted. Even she knew that there are times when you have to admit defeat.

For tonight the war was over; damage assessment and rebuilding would have to wait until the morning. In the meantime I had to deaden my mind; enter the greatest mind deadener of them all: the television. As I lay there and watched with my grandparents, I once again became lost in another world, one that was not full of frustration, illness and loneliness. The daily trials of soap characters seemed almost pathetic in comparison to the desperation I was experiencing. I went to bed that night more uncertain of my future than ever. I did have a glimmer of peace though; at least I may be allowed to stop fighting quite so hard. Perhaps I was finally beginning to be heard?

With my life reaching crisis point, a solution was required.

Something had to give. If it were not my health and consequent sanity, then it would have to be school. The next day was spent discussing my options. Dropping out of school altogether was very appealing in that it would totally stop the pressure. However, what would I do with the hour or so of energy a day that I did have? Leaving school would mean that I would go from having little contact with the outside world to having absolutely none. Although there was a part of me that liked the idea of further withdrawing from life as I had come to know it, the thought of spending even more time alone with my growing depression was rather frightening. I therefore chose a compromise.

The best option seemed to be for me to continue with one of my three A-levels (economics, business studies and history) for the remaining half of the year, and then to repeat the first year of the other two subjects the following year. After that, in my third year, I would then do the final year of all three subjects. This way I would still get my A-levels, but I would be able to gradually build up my strength. It seemed like the ideal solution.

The next step was to work out the funding, for my grandmother had only budgeted to pay two years' fees. The school was contacted, and it was agreed that I could have the final year at half price, for I had been using almost no facilities, and I was a potentially promising student that they did not appear to want to lose.

The next six months of my life were spent basically as a prisoner of illness who had a one-hour exercise period of school each day. I never went out, saw friends, or did anything social, that is apart from have regular appointments with an increasingly baffled Dr. Mansfield. The months blurred into one and almost nothing of interest happened. In fact, I may as well have been dead. In many ways I was. The only emotion I really felt was depression. There were, however, a couple of events that stood out from the blackness, but only because they were particularly dark.

One Sunday night, when I was visiting home, I was lying in bed trying to get to sleep. This was something that I found surprisingly difficult considering how tired I always felt. As I lay there hugging my duvet and extra blankets tight, pretending they could protect me from the pains of my life, my left leg suddenly jerked as though electricity had been passed through it. My heart skipped a beat. What the hell had just happened? I was used to feeling shaky, but this was different.

For a few moments I started to panic, terrified at what might be

41

going on. But, after a time I did manage to calm myself, deciding it was just a freak occurrence and I once more tried to fall asleep. While I worked to relax and daydream, it suddenly happened again. If I had felt out of control of my health in the past, this was at a new level. My body was moving without my volition. I became increasingly anxious as it continued to happen. Soon my arms were also jerking involuntarily. That is to say nothing of my heart palpitating and the fact that I was totally freezing, despite the extra blankets wrapped all around me. Even the dull light shining under the door from the corridor outside was aggravating me. Just being alive was becoming agony.

I was soon so scared by my out of control body that I couldn't bear to be alone any longer and I screamed out for help. As Mum rushed to my side, I was starting to shake uncontrollably. She was visibly shocked by the state she found me in and was desperately trying to decide whether to call an ambulance or not. Yet, despite the clear horror of what was happening, there didn't seem to be any point. What could a paramedic do anyway? The several doctors that I had seen all appeared equally lost. In the end Mum just tried the best she could to comfort me and get me to think happy thoughts. This was almost impossible. The last nine months of my life had been just pure illness. It felt like there was no hope. With Mum sitting by my side for most of the night, I did eventually fall asleep and the shaking slowly settled. I wish I could say the same for the rest of the volatility around me.

My sister had again just been committed to a mental hospital, on this occasion for serious violence towards our Mum and grandmother, along with trying to overdose on paracetamol. My mum and stepfather were also in the process of trying to sell our home as part of their most recent attempt to divorce. What did I feel? To be honest I felt only one added emotion beyond my already severe depression: I felt emotionally sick. I was sick of the constant suffering. I was sick of my family. I was sick of being behind at school. I was sick of having no friends. I was sick of the constant sleeping. And, worst of all, I was sick of being sick.

CHAPTER 8: A LITTLE LIGHT BURNING IN THE DARKNESS (SUMMER 1997 TO SUMMER 1998)

What am I supposed to say when I'm not all right?
What am I supposed to say when I'm just fine?
Tomorrow has gone away again, but I'm still looking for today.
Looking For Today (written by Alex Howard, recorded by Sugarkane for "Star Destroyer EP")

By the summer little had changed with my health, but there was a tiny light beginning to penetrate the darkness of my days. Tom and Dale, who were in the band that had started just as I got ill, were playing music together again. With Nick sacked, they now had Tom's girlfriend, Claire, playing the drums, and they had already been into the studio to make a mini-album. One night Dale called me up on the telephone and offered me the job of lead guitarist for the new band. I think I genuinely smiled that night for the first time in nearly a year.

Band practice on Sunday mornings became like a weekly release from prison. To have the opportunity to make music with friends again was just incredible. I would spend the entire week dreaming about those two hours while Claire's family went to football and we piled around the drum kit in her bedroom. I once again finally had something to live for. After lengthy discussions, we decided to call the band Sugarkane, quite ironic considering I was the only person I knew who was unable to eat sugar!

Being in the band also meant that I had some contact with the outside world that was more than just five one-hour classes feeling ill at school each week. Towards the end of the summer, every so often I even started to have Tom, Dale and Claire, along with a few of their friends, around for a couple of hours in the evening. As at school, I pretended that all was well with my health and that the only problem was that I needed a lot of sleep. I even joked about it. I believed that no one could understand the hell that my world had become, and so I didn't give anyone the chance. I also feared scaring people away. Having spent the last year with only my neurosis and depression to keep me company, I had come to realise what a precious commodity friends were.

In addition to pretending to be something that I was not, I also convinced my mum to provide alcohol for everyone. Being ill, I felt I had to buy love more than ever. Because I felt spaced out and like I was drunk the whole time, drinking alcohol no longer appealed to me. Having grown up around alcoholism and seen the transformations that it created in the people I loved, I also perceived it more as an abused drug than as a way of having fun. Witnessing the way that many of my peers drank to the point of vomiting, there appeared to be little evidence that I had been mistaken. No one had any idea that this was how I really felt, and I was relieved that my health gave me an excuse to keep things this way.

As a consequence of my continuing illness, I had been living at my grandparents for the last year. It had been the easiest option, as my grandmother had effectively been my carer, along with driving me to and from school and cooking meals. However, I missed being at home and the added independence it gave me. Although I had been thinking about moving home for a while, life at my grandparents reached an end for me quite abruptly when one day my sister moved back in with my grandparents after being discharged from hospital.

Watching the way my grandmother interacted with George, I intuitively knew that, despite George being the one that everyone saw as ill, my grandmother's behaviour with her was contributing massively to the resultant problems. Unable to witness this without voicing my opinions, my grandmother and I had an argument and I decided that I had had enough, I called my stepfather to come and collect my things and drive me home. Although it was a relief to be home once again, I was very grateful for the invaluable support my grandmother had given me over the past year.

By the end of the summer, after many weeks' anticipation, I played my first gig with Sugarkane. It was by far the most physically exhausting thing I had done since I had first been ill, but I didn't care; playing music was the only love I had left. All I had to do was stand on stage for thirty minutes and I would get to experience what I had always dreamed of. The gig was for a group of Italian students who were visiting Dorking. It was hardly Wembley Stadium, but as far as we were concerned it could have been. For the rest of the band, the only fear that they had was making a mistake. With the anxiety I had about passing out or being too ill to play, this was the last thing on my mind.

I spent the day of the gig lying on the sofa at home trying to lose myself in the television. I had recently discovered the video box set of "Billy Connolly's World Tour of Australia," and was watching the entire series for about the seventh time. It fitted my requirements for escapism perfectly: it was full of optimism, humour and a hot country the other side of the world. For a few hours I was able to enter a land of happiness.

My latest problem was that my right arm ached, meaning playing the guitar was even more of an effort than usual. I feared that it might also mean I would be unable to play the gig that night. If only I hadn't practiced so much the previous week, I cursed myself. Visions of being unable to play, along with how ill I might feel when I got back after the show, ran through my mind right up until I met the others at the venue. Thankfully, my determination outweighed any attempts by my brutal illness to jeopardise what we had all worked so hard for.

As I sat in the car with the rest of the band afterwards, I felt more excitement than I had done since I had first become sick. The gig had been a huge success and we had been invited back again the next year. We were even paid £50. Considering the dozens of hours of rehearsals it wasn't much. However, I reasoned that we had played for thirty minutes and, with the money split four ways, that meant we were each worth £25 an hour! A few weeks later we had a one-day session at a recording studio. I couldn't wait. One of my childhood dreams was about to come true.

Yet, as my illness now guaranteed, my experience was severely contaminated. Being in the studio meant that I had to spend twelve hours out of bed, and therefore my strategically placed periods of sleep, which I usually needed to get through a day just resting on the sofa, had to be missed. By the time I got home in the evening I was beyond exhausted, but I didn't care; I had my first demo tape! Whatever had happened in the last year, at least no one could take that away from me.

Over the next few days, in comparing what I had actually done to what I had believed my physical limits to be, I started to feel a new level of confidence. If I could do that once, then why not again? It seemed that the more I enjoyed what I was doing, despite my intense dizziness, fatigue and muscle aches, the more suffering I could tolerate. The life of doing nothing had been all I could do for now. However, except for a couple of hours with the band each week, I was bored. Totally, and utterly, bored. Bored to death, almost literally. I no longer cared so much if I went to bed completely knackered; I was used to it anyway. I needed some kind of a life again, even if it meant I would spend every minute of every day feeling ill.

With the new school year having soon started again, I did once more feel like I was competing in a daily marathon. But, it did still feel better than the life of loneliness that I had experienced the previous year. The growing success of Sugarkane undoubtedly made my survival easier.

By the fifth week of term we had our first pub gig, which was mentioned on local radio and featured in the local paper. My enthusiasm for our music, along with a burning desire to succeed, made me a great promoter, and I spent as much time at school as I could publicising our coming event. My teachers couldn't understand how I could find the energy for music when I was struggling with a few hours of school a day, I couldn't have cared less that they didn't realise I was still sleeping much of the day. As far as I was concerned, appearing to be a rebel added to my rockstar image.

On the evening of the gig, a number of people I knew from St. John's turned out, proving my promotion efforts had in fact all been worth it; or so I thought. Only over eighteens were allowed entry and none of them were (thankfully the bouncers never questioned my age, as I was still only just seventeen). To say I wasn't very popular in class the following Monday is an understatement, but at least I could continue to enthuse that we were the best live band around and no one could say anything to the contrary!

My only regret, the one thing that hung like a black cloud over the whole day, that was still a storm brewing over my whole life, was my illness. I spent the entire evening in a state of fear, and at times terror, of passing out and not having enough energy to get through the gig. Needing to spend almost the whole of the following day in bed struggling to recover just added to my frustration.

By the end of the school year little with my health had changed; I still felt extremely ill every day. Thankfully, despite my inner stagnation, Sugarkane were continuing to grow in stature. Tom, Dale, Claire and I had played a couple of gigs in London, recorded another mini-album, and truly believed that by the end of the summer we might get a record deal. We decided to dedicate the summer holidays to rehearsing, recording and gigging, in an attempt to realise this dream.

However, although the band was clearly still a flame burning strongly in the darkness of my life, it was not enough to illuminate the blackness left by my state of mind. My depression was in many ways still building. With every extra month of ME, I was developing a further looming sense of fear as to what a future of illness might entail. I even started to wonder if I would ever get better. Such thoughts petrified me. I couldn't even bear considering how horrific an existence spending the rest of my life ill would be.

In the midst of this bizarre contrast of musical passion and deep depression, I had what at that point was one of the most powerful experiences of my life. I went to see Ravi Panniah, an iridologist, medical guru, and an all round pretty amazing guy. My uncle, Iain, who had been seriously impressed by Ravi's abilities, had arranged the appointment, and was also paying for it, as, unlike Dr. Mansfield's consultations, it would not be covered under my medical insurance.

"I'll be incredibly surprised if you don't get a diagnosis," Iain had encouraged me a couple of days before, going on to explain to me how Ravi used the eye to diagnose what was happening in the body. In hearing this I have to confess I was rather sceptical. By this time I had been under Dr. Mansfield for eighteen months and witnessed only very marginal improvement. I had also seen a number of other practitioners, including a homeopath and nutritionist, with equally poor results. I had been let down too many times and I was slowly losing my faith. It seemed far too simple for someone to be able to just look into my eyes and tell me what was wrong with me.

Thankfully, this occasion was different. This time I got what all ME sufferers crave, the thing that most would give anything for: I actually got a proper diagnosis. What's more, this time it was something a lot more useful than, "I must confess that ME is the most likely explanation."

CHAPTER 9: A GENIUS MIRACLE WORKER TRIES HIS MAGIC (SUMMER 1998)

Do not fear to be eccentric in opinion, for every opinion now accepted was once eccentric.
Bertrand Russell

It was on a hot summer day that Mum and I embarked on our journey to Ravi's practice in Islington. Before being ill I had always loved being out in the sun, but these days I just found it drained away precious energy. With a travel time of an hour and a half each way, I knew that I would really be battling by the end.

As the train pulled away from Dorking station, my initial scepticism about iridology being such a simple form of diagnosis began to give way to excitement. Maybe this really would be the turning point, I wondered to myself. Perhaps I really would once again be able to live a normal life. I began to have visions of playing golf that summer. My God, how amazing it would be to spend time with friends doing real physical exercise, I yearned. What if I was even healthy enough to go on holiday? I hadn't been away for two years. I might even be well enough to date girls again! While I imagined an alternative future to that based on my current experience, I couldn't resist a little smile.

"Please God, let this be it," I said aloud, but really talking to myself.

"I really hope it is," said Mum, with a look of true compassion in her eyes, "You deserve it more than anyone."

If only life was run on such criteria, I thought to myself.

As was inevitable when I considered the way my life could be, I felt a sense of jealousy of my peers. Had I not suffered enough? Had I not already done everything that I could to get better? I had stuck to the diets. I had rested as much as I could. I had even tolerated that counsellor for two sessions. It just didn't seem fair.

Yet, somewhere inside of me I knew that there must be a reason for what was happening. I somehow knew that I must have been going through hell for some reason other than just to get burnt. After all, if that were the case I was burnt out anyway. What if there was another part of my being that needed burning or changing? However, such an idea was of little interest to me when I wanted back my old life so badly.

Once Mum and I arrived in Islington, having negotiated the London Underground with my fragile body, we fought our way through the crowds and market stalls of Chapel Market to reach "Insight Care" where Ravi worked. Stepping inside, and leaving behind the hustle and bustle of midweek London, provided welcome refreshment. A mini-waterfall dripping in one of the corners added to my rejuvenation, giving the sense of entering an oasis in the middle of the city.

While Mum and I waited for my appointment, we took a seat in the waiting area and flicked through the magazines. We saw whom we assumed to be Ravi come out of one of the consultation rooms several times and instruct staff about various treatments that patients needed to have prepared. To say he radiated health and vitality was a major understatement. His dark skin looked perfect, and his moustache appeared as though the hairs had been measured before being trimmed it was so precise. I was later to discover that Ravi lived on three hours sleep a night and ran seven miles every morning. He was certainly not your average middle-aged consultant!

Apart from having clearly created optimum health in himself, Ravi had a number of areas of professional expertise. To start with, he was a practitioner of conventional medicine. However, he was also much, much, more than this. In addition to using the iris as his main source of diagnosis, Ravi treated his patients using traditional medicine in the form of vitamins and minerals, and alternative techniques such as homeopathy, herbs, and acupuncture. Quite remarkably, Iain had explained to me that Ravi would not even ask what was wrong with me. That was for him to find out. To me this was quite novel. It was also rather amusing sitting in the waiting room wondering whether he would get it right!

After a while, Ravi introduced himself and invited us into his office, which could easily be distinguished from a conventional doctor's surgery by the presence of reference books on both Eastern and Western medicine. As we sat down, Ravi gave a brief explanation of what he did, and then used a magnifying glass to look in my eye. A few moments later, he leant back in his chair and described in detail every single one of the symptoms I was experiencing. He was unbelievably accurate, down to minute details such as what time I would wake up at in the night feeling ill, when my symptoms had started (to the month), and the anxiety that I was experiencing as a consequence. He even knew I had eaten chicken for dinner the night before!

For a few moments I was rendered speechless by Ravi's demonstration of his abilities. I just could not understand how he had obtained so much information from looking in my eyes. However, within a couple of minutes my shock had developed into the most incredible relief.

Someone finally knew what was wrong with me! Of course much more important than describing my symptoms, which would only have made Ravi a magician, he also had the reasons why. Most importantly, he had a treatment plan.

As I continued to sit there in a state of awe, Ravi described how initially I had had a viral infection, similar to glandular fever, which had wiped me out. Resultant from this, I had developed hypoglycaemia (low blood sugar), which was why I woke up in the middle of the night feeling dizzy and spaced out, i.e. because my blood sugar levels were too low. He explained that due to my pancreas struggling, my body was not recovering from the hypoglycaemia, as it should be doing. Consequent to my blood sugar levels fluctuating, my adrenal glands were getting continually burnt out as they worked to compensate. The overall state of anxiety created by my situation was also not helping.

Ravi next explained how he was going to assist my body in healing itself. My pancreas, which he saw as the source of my weaknesses, was to be treated using homeopathic remedies, and I was also to take several mineral solutions and other vitamins to support my immune system and general physical health. Within eight months (two total blood changes) my energy levels should be back to normal, and Ravi could see no reason why I would not make a full recovery. I could barely believe my ears! I dreamed that it now might finally be time, after two years of chronic illness, for my life to be returned.

Although Ravi had created a powerful impression on me, on the way home a part of me was still a bit sceptical. Could it really be this easy for my life to be transformed? Could two years of chronic illness just be due to a viral infection and a weak pancreas? But, despite my concerns, within a few days I had thrown caution to the wind and told everyone I knew that I would make a total recovery within the next eight months. All I had to do was take a homeopathic remedy three times a day, drink a foul-tasting mineral solution each morning, swallow a few vitamin supplements, and I would once again have a normal life.

Soon summer holidays had arrived and I had band practice four mornings a week. With school no longer on the agenda for two months, I also had time for more of a social life. Some evenings I would go out to the pub with the other band members, and I always had my best friend, the television, if I got bored. Within a few weeks of the summer beginning, promotional efforts were paying off and Sugarkane had a number of major gigs booked. One was headlining at the Mean Fiddler in London (the main venue of the company that organises a number of the big summer festivals such as Reading). Another was the one gig that we had always wanted: the newly refurbished Dorking Halls (the biggest venue near where I grew up, holding 600+ people).

Sugarkane were also going into the studio again. This time we were entering the world of digital recording, meaning that I would be able to record all the guitar parts. This boosted my ego no end. With the catchy new songs we were working on, and the coming gigs and studio time, things for the band were looking better than ever. However, there was one major problem: Tom, Dale and Claire were all going to university in September, that was, unless we got a record deal. This was our ultimate goal, and it was where we set our sights. With this new vision of a career in music, my life became a lot more bearable. I still had to sleep for several hours every afternoon, and I still felt ill all of the time, but at least I had the daily pleasure of fulfilling my love of writing and playing music.

At my second appointment to see Ravi I had another extraordinary experience, although this time it was a different kind of extraordinary. While Ravi was treating me he commented that Nick McCave, the lead guitarist from The Verve, had the next appointment and that he would introduce us. Although Iain had told me that Ravi had a number of famous clients, I had never expected that I would get to meet any of them!

As I sat there in the waiting room, reading the latest issue of "Guitarist" and waiting for my homeopathic remedies to be prepared, who should walk in and sit right next to me but Nick McCave. Knowing that I was the closest I had ever been to someone famous, my mind sped up in an attempt to find an appropriate introduction. I wondered whether I should introduce myself and ask for an autograph, or should I play it cool and just wait for Ravi to do the honours? Perhaps I should think of something witty and funny to say and try to make Nick McCave laugh? While my mind weighed up the pros and cons of each option, I slowly turned the pages of my magazine, attempting to look as though I was reading it. However, the longer I waited, the more awkward it started to feel; any chance of sounding spontaneous was gone. As I continued struggling to resolve the inner civil war that was brewing in my mind, Ravi appeared. I breathed a sigh of relief, knowing that everything would be done for me.

"Hi Nick," said Ravi, as he collected some notes from the

51

receptionist, "This is Alex, he's a guitarist as well."

"Hi," said Nick McCave as he shook my hand, before following Ravi into the consultation room.

"Hi," I mumbled as they walked away, unable to think of anything more to say. Before I knew it, the door had closed behind them and my big chance was gone. "You moron," I said to myself, "You just blew the opportunity of a lifetime." As I collected my remedies and made my way home, I continued beating myself up for ruining my big chance. Sugarkane could have been the support band on The Verve's next tour!

A week later my inner turmoil had settled and my experience was now just a great memory. I was also surprised to hear that The Verve had just announced their split. So much for being their support band.

At my third appointment I got another big surprise. Call it a coincidence if you like, but who should have an adjacent appointment to me this time but Richard Ashcroft, the lead singer of The Verve. This time I didn't get a chance to be introduced, but I didn't care. As far as I was concerned I was on my way to socialising with the rich and famous!

Unfortunately, despite my celebrity encounters, by the middle of August my health was declining again. I was struggling with persistent tonsillitis (which I refused to take antibiotics for due to the risks of recreating a candida overgrowth), and the result was that I was even more wiped out than usual. Even though I had two years of practice, I still had a hard time accepting such dips in my health, especially when they were so deep.

I wondered why the benefits of Ravi's treatment were not showing. Why was I feeling worse rather than better? Something was obviously not right. Ravi said that I had to give it time, but I did not feel like I had time. Band practice was once more becoming a major effort, and again I was struggling with my schoolwork (which I was supposed to be completing before school recommenced). The lightness of the start of the summer was rapidly giving way to a feeling of impending doom with a new school year lingering. Most frightening of all was that once again I was going to have to survive without the cushion of playing music with my friends twice a week, for the dreamed of record deal was looking more and more like just that, a dream.

One day that summer which particularly stood out from the rest was Thursday 20th August 1998. It was the day of A-level results and, if had I not been ill, the day I would have officially finished school. It was also the night of Sugarkane's headlining gig at the Mean Fiddler. Due to my continuing acute tonsillitis I had missed several vital band practices, and I had heard, learnt and played one of the new songs for that night only the day before. I had only survived the rehearsal by sleeping in the middle.

With my again declining health, the overwhelming anxieties of the past were back with more brutal strength than ever. The relentless old records of me being too ill to survive even my pathetic existence seemed to be on a never-ending loop in my mind. After all, I would cleverly remind myself, we were not due on stage until 10:15, and I would normally be asleep by that time. I would then remember the months on end that I had spent in bed in the past when I had overdone it and how now, before I even played the gig, I was on the verge of such an episode. I just wished I could be free from the monotonous anxieties.

Sound-check started at 5:00, but there was no way that I was going to be able to last from 3:00 in the afternoon (it would take two hours to get to the venue) until 1:00 the next morning. An added problem was the fact that Mum did not like driving in London due to her limited eyesight, and I did not feel well enough to take the train. For a while it looked like I had no way of getting to the gig, but thankfully a solution came in the form of my aunt and uncle who offered to drive me there a few hours before I was due on stage. It was at times like these, in the midst of despair, that I was truly thankful for the kindness of others.

As I dragged myself out of bed in the late afternoon, I felt very determined, praying that I would somehow get through. I hoped that if I did make it, the consequences would not be too severe. When I arrived at the venue, everyone in the band was in a jovial mood after exam results, especially Claire who had come top of her school by scoring an unbeatable four A's.

Having congratulated the others on their results, I took a much-needed rest before the doors opened. Lying on one of the sofas in the backstage area, I wondered to myself, where would I be in a year's time? Would every day still be a constant battle with the world around me? Would I still be seriously ill, or would I by some miracle be well enough to go to university? Little did I know that the next year was going to be the most important of my life; I was going to face the ultimate choice: live or die?

After a while, the two bands before us took to the stage. We were relieved to discover that, despite their superior experience, our headlining position was justified. When our time came, having not sound-checked my guitar, only played one of the songs for the first time the day before, and not even knowing if I would get through the gig, I walked out on stage.

Our opening song, named "Love Letters for Edward," was one of my favourites. It was really hard hitting with a great lead guitar part that I always enjoyed playing, when I was not full of anxiety, fear and illness anyway. The crowd seemed quite static, but we gave it everything we could. Despite the adrenaline rush of performing, my fears were still lingering. The bright lights glaring in my eyes were certainly not helping. Something, as always, wasn't right. I tried to ignore it and push it out of my mind. Yet, it wasn't working, the fear was still building. What did I think I was playing at? I might be running on adrenaline for now, but that could only last for so long.

Tom started the second song, "Caroline and Me," and as the rest of us came crashing in together I felt like I was going to fall. It was developing into a real effort just to stay on my feet. I had my most difficult guitar part towards the end of this song and I was going to need to access all my abilities. I had written my solo purely for showmanship. To an onlooker, my fingers would become a blur the note changes were so fast. But, if I didn't get it exactly right, the effect would be lost and I would look like an incompetent show-off. I looked over at the stage door. If I ran, I could be backstage in a matter of seconds. I would have to get round the others, but at least I wouldn't have to face these horrible feelings of dizziness.

By the time my solo was nearly upon me I had decided to stick it out, but not because I thought I could handle it. I figured that to justify my flight from the stage would be more difficult than explaining my collapsing. After all, that would be self-explanatory. I guess I had learnt very little from the hairdresser's, which didn't seem all that far away right now. I gritted my teeth and went for it, resigning myself to the fact that I could collapse any minute.

As Tom hung on the last note of the chorus and we went into the bridge before my guitar solo, my heart skipped several beats. Before I knew it, Claire was shaking the drum kit with the intensity of her drum-fill that cued my solo. I only had a few seconds left. Almost without thinking about it, I stepped forward into the spotlight, hit my boost pedal with my right foot and began my ride of the wave of musical passion. Lifting my head towards the ceiling in classic rock fashion, I let the music take over and for a few moments I entered another place. As my solo reached its climax, I lowered my glance and gazed at the crowd. To my massive relief, despite the haziness of my vision, I noticed some approving faces. For a second I relaxed inside, but, before I knew it, my anxiety was back and I had the next song to think about.

For nearly an hour the four of us continued to entertain. Somehow I hit all my cues and remembered all my vocal harmonies. And, despite my internal nightmare, we still created some magical musical moments that night. When we eventually left the stage to rapturous applause and cheers from the crowd, much to my surprise I was still standing. I thankfully also just had enough drive left in me to get home and into bed.

Just in time for our stint in the recording studio my tonsillitis did eventually subside, and fortunately there was no long-term damage to my health after the gig. I was therefore back from being very seriously ill, to being just seriously ill. Thank God for small mercies.

A few weeks later was Dorking Halls; our second to last gig together. It was in many ways the night that I achieved one of my greatest ambitions. I had walked past the building and dreamed of performing there every day for four years on my way home from secondary school, ever since I had got my first guitar. It was undisputedly the pinnacle of local venues. Many of my family and old friends were there to share our supposed night of glory and the gig itself went well, apart form a couple of hairy moments: one where I got my foot caught on a guitar lead and nearly fell over and another when I broke a string on my guitar. Yet, once again, the night was still overshadowed by my health problems.

The next night, a pub gig in Crawley, was to be the last time Sugarkane ever played together. The dreamed of record contract had never materialised, and so Tom, Dale and Claire all went to their chosen universities. It was over. The little light illuminating the darkness of my life was extinguished. My time had finally come. No longer was I going to be able to my live as a victim of life. The pain was now great enough for me to let go of whom I took to be me, and embark on a dramatic journey of personal transformation. After eighteen years of intermittent hell, I was finally about to wake up.

CHAPTER 10: THE LIGHT GOES OUT, ANYONE OUT THERE? (AUTUMN 1998)

Frodo: I wish none of this had happened.
Gandalf: So do all who live to see such times, but that is not for
them to decide. All we have to decide is what to do with the time
that is given to us.
The Lord of the Rings

September saw me back at school, and once again facing my daily hell of classes, sleep, homework, sleep, television, and then, of course, more sleep. The monotony was monumental, and I no longer had music to escape to. Just to top things off, I had the most important exams of my life at the end of the year. If I failed these, then I would also lose the opportunity to go to university and escape the additional horror of living in the middle of my family war-zone. I had no idea how I would physically survive looking after myself if I got to university, but one thing was for sure: if I was forced to live much longer where I was I would be committing slow suicide anyway.

There appeared to be no way out of my daily hell. I had thought that this time with Ravi I really had found the answers. Once again I had been wrong. By this stage I had been to almost a dozen different practitioners, I had totally changed my diet, I had read several books on healing, and I had even tried practising a form of Tai Chi (called qigong). For some mysterious reason my body was failing to respond to everything I did. Each time something else didn't work was like another nail in my coffin, the disappointments seemed to get harder and harder to bear.

Within a month of being back at school, continuing with my life as it was finally became impossible. The path of hoping I had been so desperately following reached a dead-end. For the first time I seriously started to entertain the idea that I might never recover. I had already spent two years fighting ME with absolutely nothing to show for my efforts, apart from even more pain and depression. In many ways my health was worse now than it had been at the start of my illness. At least then I had had my mind. I could on longer ever remember how it felt to be healthy.

One cold Thursday night I was lying on the living room sofa at home flicking through the channels on the television, searching for something that might lift my sinking mood. It seemed that on this night I had fallen even lower than usual, for even the television could not stop me from dropping further. Why? I kept asking myself. Why me? Why had this happened to me? Why was my life so full of suffering? Why did nothing work? Why was the world around me such a mess? The further I fell, the more scared I became. The more scared I became, the more I started to question. Why? Why? Why?

Yet, while I continued to lie at the mercy of my increasingly twisted mind, a part of me was still searching for a way out. Despite the clear magnitude of my problems, it continued to insist that there had to be something I could do. As I racked my brain, searching my history for solutions, one person's name kept popping up, my uncle, Iain. I remembered times when he had powerfully impacted upon my life in the past.

Mum had never been wealthy, and despite her working two or three jobs at a time keeping us comfortable, there was rarely the money for luxuries. While Iain and I were kicking a football around one afternoon after a family lunch, a rare treat for me due to my lack of a father figure, I made a passing comment about his designer trainers. The next day my grandmother telephoned to say that he had left me £50 to buy a pair for myself. I was normally lucky if I was allowed to spend £30 on a pair of shoes. By having a "cool" pair of trainers, my popularity at school actually increased for several days. The gift was totally unexpected, and I had done nothing to earn it. I was very unused to such acts of generosity.

On another occasion a few years later, we were walking past Woolworth's after a similar family occasion. Iain spontaneously took my sister and I in and told us each to pick any three tapes we wanted. I remember distinctly to this day the privilege I felt. After some tough decisions, based on what at that time was a very limited knowledge of music, I chose Genesis- We Can't Dance, Queen- Greatest Hits 2, and Now 20 (a compilation album). Throughout my childhood I treasured those three tapes like they were the crown jewels. In many ways to me they were, for they were the birth of my love of modern music. However, Iain's impact on my relationship with music did not end here.

Within a year or so of being introduced to the likes of Genesis and Queen, Dale (bass guitar and main songwriter in Sugarkane) and I got talking in English lessons at school. In the middle of returning the rolled up clumps of paper thrown at us from the back of the class by the "cool" kids, I was rapidly educated in the ways of alternative rock music. Because of my mother being a piano teacher, from a young age I had studied classical music and was well educated in playing the piano and trumpet. However, my interest had wavered, and after having to give up the trumpet due to its creating pressure on my weakened eardrums, I had started studying the acoustic guitar. The more Dale introduced me to various kinds of rock music, the less I cared about playing classically. I had to have an electric guitar and sound like my new idols. It felt like my life depended on it.

The guitar I desired was going to cost £200, and as there was no way that I would be able to afford an amplifier as well I was planning to plug it into my stereo. I was so in love with my future companion that I visited the local music shop as a weekly pilgrimage every Friday after school. However, despite having spent six months saving as much as I could of my pocket money, and the £7.50 a week that I got for delivering papers (terrible money for getting up at 6.00 six mornings a week), I was still only half way there.

One Friday afternoon, just as I was finishing dinner at my grandparents, Iain phoned to say that he had bought the guitar for me, along with a proper amplifier. I was totally blown away and virtually speechless. To say that the gift was out of the blue is a massive understatement. I could not even remember telling Iain I had been saving for it. The next day, when I went to collect my new friend from the music shop, was probably my happiest childhood experience.

As I considered just how much Iain had impacted upon my life up until now, I desperately hoped that he might be able to use some similar magic to help lift me from my growing depression and despair. It would be a challenge though. Things were so unlike the past. Even when I had called Iain several months previously and he had recommended Ravi to me I had been in a very different place to now. Back then I had been frustrated, and getting better was the most important thing in my life. Now it was the only thing. An old proverb says:

When the pupil is ready, the teacher will appear.

Well, I was ready. I was more lost than I had known it was possible to be. I dialled Iain's number.

Iain answered the telephone in his usual direct manner and asked how I was. This was a question I hated having to answer. I tended to just say I was fine and change the subject, not really wanting to consider the reality of what was actually happening to me. However, tonight the horror of what I was experiencing was too in my face to ignore. It was, after all, also the reason I was calling. I took a deep breath and told Iain the truth: I hated my life.

Iain's response was very different to what I was used to. On the rare occasions that I did tell people how much I was struggling, I would generally get a reply in the realms of, "Oh, that's terrible, you must be so fed up," or the equally popular, "You poor thing." However, Iain was coming from a very different place. It was obvious to him that sympathy wouldn't change things. What I needed was to hear life's wake up call. After all, the universe couldn't have been screaming much louder. What was to follow was without doubt the most important conversation of my life. As I was to discover a bit further down the line, it probably also saved it.

"I have a question for you. How badly do you want to change things?" Iain asked. "On a scale of one to ten, ten being you would do anything, where do you rate yourself?" To me this initially sounded like a silly question; I was obviously a ten. However, upon closer reflection I guessed there were a few things I would hesitate to try, such as being a subject for dangerous experimental drugs.

"A nine or a ten," I offered. "I would do almost anything."

"Interesting," Iain said. At this point my mind started to race. Interesting? What did that mean? This had to be leading somewhere. "Are you up for a little exercise?" Iain questioned.

"Sure," I replied, intrigued at how it was going to help me.

"This evening, over the next day or two, or whenever you get the chance, make a list of all the things you think you could do to get better. Include anything and everything that comes, just letting your mind flow without judging. When you have finished, make a list of all the things that make you worse."

"I'll do it right away and phone you back," I offered, still feeling intrigued, and also sensing Iain didn't want me to ask questions for now.

As soon as I put the phone down, I grabbed a pen and some paper and set to work on my exercise. I began with the list of things I could do to get better. First, I put down continuing with my "special diet" and seeing Ravi. I then added re-starting the qigong for, even though I had discarded it over a year ago, I figured it might still have some benefit. Other possibilities I included were yoga, meditation, psychotherapy, and also reading some books on ME for extra information (producing the list was making me realise just how little I really knew). As far as the things that made me worse, I did have stress and school, but it felt like it was more life in general that was the problem.

Once I had finished I phoned Iain back and shared my lists with him.

"How many hours a day do you spend doing the things that you yourself have listed as being beneficial?" was Iain's response.

"Erm, well, I do the diet already; as for the others I guess not much, but I don't really have the time. I only just have enough energy for school," I replied.

"So, you said you are a nine or a ten, but devote almost none of your time to things that you yourself think might help? I'm not being judgmental, but you asked for my advice. If you really are a nine or ten, then surely you should be utilising your time more appropriately?" Iain suggested.

Iain had a point, if I really wanted my life to change more than anything, then why was I not using my time in a way that was consistent with this? Yet I wondered, could it really be that simple? It wasn't like I hadn't been trying to get better. I was also feeling a bit like I was getting the blame for my life not changing. It was hardly my fault, I told myself, unaware of the massive difference between blame and responsibility.

"I really struggle with school as it is," I explained. "I don't have a spare minute in the day because every moment I have is spent trying to study or rest."

"But if you want to get better badly enough you will have to make the time. You're not going to die from what you have got. Most people in your position resign themselves to the practices of conventional medicine, but, as you know, they don't get very far. If it is important enough to you, then you will have to decide to be different," was Iain's reply.

"I guess," I said, wondering; did Iain really believe I had it within me to turn my life around? He certainly had my curiosity.

Having got the leverage necessary, Iain went on.

"How many hours television a day are you watching at the moment?"

"Erm, about six," I eventually replied in a rather embarrassed voice, shocked myself at the figure I had reached after counting the various hours throughout the day I spent lying on the sofa or in bed numbing my brain.

"But it helps me relax and removes the boredom of just lying down," I ventured, sensing that one of the small crutches left in my wretched life was under attack.

"That may be so, but it is still six hours a day which you could spend doing other things," Iain pointed out.

"But the time I spend watching television I am just lying down with no energy to do anything apart from stare at the screen," I tried, fearing I was losing.

"Watching television is not necessarily harmful, but it will not benefit your recovery. How about reading a book? You did yourself say that you need more information on recovering from ME," responded Iain.

"Er, I guess that could help, but I wouldn't know where to start," I continued with the excuses.

"Well I can help you with books to read, and although it's not going to directly improve your health, it could be a source of information that provides the answers you need. I'm not saying that you have to give up watching television altogether, but you could at least cut down the number of hours and reallocate the rest of your time," Iain suggested.

"How about the other things on the list, the yoga and the qigong?" Iain continued.

"Well I did do the qigong for a couple of weeks, but it made no difference. Anyway, if I have almost no energy to start with, what is the point in wasting it exercising?" I replied.

"If you haven't really tried it properly, how do you know?" was Iain's answer. "I know that after a long day at the office sometimes I feel really drained, but I always feel better after going to yoga or qigong. Anyway, is it not the theory of qigong that it increases your energy?"

"But the way I feel is not like normal tiredness," I attempted to explain.

In some ways my situation still felt useless, and I was trying to convince myself how much easier it would be to wait for someone else to change my life. At the same time, I was also becoming rather stunned at how little I was actively doing to transform something that Iain quite clearly believed I could.

"It may be the case that your tiredness is different, and I'm not suggesting that you go for hours at once, but even five minutes a day could lead to obvious benefits," Iain offered.

"I suppose I could try," I replied tentatively, far from being convinced that qigong was going to change my life. Yet, I kept reminding myself that I had said I was a nine or a ten and how inconsistent the way I lived was with that. If I wanted to get better more than anything, then perhaps I was going to have to do something dramatic about it.

"And the meditation and the psychotherapy, do you think you could find time in your busy schedule for those?" Iain continued with a playful tone in his voice, lightening the situation.

"I could give it a go," I replied, beginning to feel more determined.

After all, I reminded myself, meditation is hardly an exhausting practice!

The next half-hour or so continued with Iain guiding me in outlining a strategy by which I could do what so many infinitely more educated people before me had failed at: find a cure for ME. As exciting as my new challenge was though, a large part of me was still screaming to ignore Iain's guidance. I could feel life pulling me down a very different path to those around me, and the thought of becoming even more shut off from my peers was a scary one. Most people already thought I was insane by not drinking alcohol and my never-ending need for sleep. Not watching television and starting to meditate and practice yoga would only add to such perceptions. However, I was also starting to realise something else: people that thought this way were perhaps not all that sane themselves.

It really began to become clear to me that even though my situation was more extreme than many people's, I was certainly not the only one who had problems. The only difference for me was that I was not going to run away from mine anymore. I also wondered, even if I was going to leave a whole load of people behind, possibly even everyone I knew, were they really the kind of people that I would choose to live with in the world of my dreams? And, despite my fears, the truth was that I also had little choice anyway. If I wanted my life to change it seemed pretty clear: I was going to have to change.

I therefore made a number of commitments to myself, so as to ensure that my new action plan became more than just a plan. Included in these was a decision to watch no more than two hours television a day, and to spend the extra four hours doing my other commitments. These were to meditate for half an hour, to do five minutes yoga and qigong, and also to look for a psychotherapist (yes, I really was willing to try anything). On top of this, I was going to use as much of my time as possible to read books about how I could change my situation.

And so, off I set on the greatest adventure of my life, not just a journey of healing as I had initially intended, but also a journey of self-discovery. I was to discover (i.e. dis-cover) my greatest fears, my true loves, and, most importantly, I was to embark on an even greater journey, the journey of real adulthood: to find out who I am and why I am really here.

CHAPTER 11: GATHERING WOOD FOR A FIRE (AUTUMN 1998 TO SPRING 1999)

It is not our abilities that show who we really are; it is our choices.
Harry Potter and the Chamber of Secrets

The first few days without television, attempting to quieten the torrents of my mind while meditating, and reading the first of hundreds of books I would read over the coming years were, in many ways, exciting. I had started to live what I would later come to call a 3D-life. I had Decided what I wanted, I had Devised a way of getting it, and most importantly of all, I was Doing it. With this new way of living, my life once again had some meaning. I had done something that few people ever do; I had finally, after so many years of hell, actually reached rock bottom. From a place as low as I had fallen, there was only one way to go, and that was up. For now my only dream was a life of health, a life where each day didn't mean a constant struggle with my own body. I had no way of knowing if my new actions would get me any closer to this dream, but I did know that I had to stand a better chance than I did watching television and waiting for someone else to change my life.

As the weeks started to merge into one another, the true immensity of my undertaking became clear. Finding a cure to an apparently incurable illness was one thing, but with only a few hours a day to devote to it, and in those hours simultaneously battling with muscles pains and intense dizziness, it was something else. Thankfully, I did rapidly develop one life-saving resource: unbeatable discipline. Whatever was happening, however I felt, I always did my meditation, yoga, qigong and reading. I lived like my life depended upon them. In many ways it did.

Despite the difficulty of keeping to my original commitments, I quickly decided to increase my efforts, and so was soon meditating for forty-five minutes a day and doing ten minutes yoga and qigong. I was also pushing myself to spend even more time reading, to the point that if I was awake I was rarely to be seen without a book in my hands. I figured that the harder I worked, the faster my life was going to change.

I took more action a couple of weeks later when I went in search of a meditation teacher. Although through meditating by myself I was already feeling calmer and sleeping more deeply, I still felt I was not benefiting as much as I could. After the failure of looking through the yellow pages and in the local paper, I had the idea of going to the local library. My persistence was rewarded when I found a flyer for a weekly meditation group, which before I knew it I had joined. A lady who worked with the teacher was a chartered psychologist, and so she was soon visiting me also. I was discovering an interesting phenomenon: when we take a small bit of truly determined action, the universe often does the rest.

My first night at the meditation group I went through my usual, "Will I be able to make it through?" thoughts. Both my legs ached and just getting out of bed prior to going was a major struggle. However, I knew that it was an important step. Taking the easy option in the short term could have meant the difference between a life of illness and a life of health. That was too big a risk to take, even if my body didn't agree.

The class was held in the living room of the teacher, Shirley O' Donoghue (now the author of "Working with Natural Energy"). Going for the first time was nerve-racking, as I had no idea what to expect. For all I knew I could have been the only normal person in a group full of nutcases. Thankfully, things started off rather tame, and there was not a VW van or a Bob Dylan record in sight. There were initially four other people in the class apart from me, and I was not even totally alienated by my being only eighteen years old, as there was also a couple in their late twenties.

The first evening was spent dowsing for "Bach Flower Remedies," which were plant extracts discovered and developed by Edward Bach in the early 1900's. They worked on the same principles as homeopathy, and had recently seen a surge in their popularity due to their being used by various famous people, including Cheri Blair.

Dowsing is something that many people are very sceptical about, and I have to confess that I was initially. In fact to be honest, I thought it a total load of rubbish. That was before I tried it for myself. Shirley explained that we were to hold our pendulums (effectively a crystal on the end of a piece of string) still and mentally ask a question. The crystal then, quite miraculously, rotated in one direction for yes, another for no, and a further direction for neutral. At first this seemed to me to be totally against scientific principles. But, in my subsequent reading I was to discover hard evidence explaining how dowsing taps into a person's unconscious mind and aura, the field of energy that surrounds the human organism. A person's aura is something that anyone studying a human being objectively can discover by feeling it with their hands (it can also be photographed using special instruments).

My weekly Thursday night sessions at the meditation group were to be the source of a lot of changes in my life over the coming year. However, the greatest source of my growth was undoubtedly the dozens of books I was reading. My uncle was the main source, but I also picked up books from the local library, Shirley and the members of my meditation group, and some books that I could find nowhere else I bought. The diversity of ideas and arguments I discovered was incredible, and also quite daunting. When confused and drawn between different viewpoints I tended to meditate on the problem, and by doing so a solution would often appear.

Despite my extensive research, I came across only a few books on ME. The ones that I was able to get hold of all said pretty much the same thing. They discussed possible causes and the available potential treatments, but the general conclusion was pretty much what my doctor had told me: there is no cure. The standard advice was to be patient and rest, and to possibly try some different complementary therapies. Something that rather concerned me was that several of the authors were actually ME sufferers who had been ill for decades and still hadn't recovered. They were hardly the role models I was searching for. I was looking for people that were experts in curing ME, not experts in living with it.

There was something unique in many of the books that I had come across by people who had recovered from other supposedly incurable illnesses such as AIDS and cancer. These people had got better and they knew why; they had all undergone a fundamental psychological/ spiritual shift. It was totally inspiring to read about people who based on modern medical "wisdom" should be either dead, or at the least severely ill and very depressed, yet had completely cured themselves and were living happy and fulfilled lives.

A powerful example was Niro Markoff Asistent, who was diagnosed as HIV positive and effectively given a death sentence. There were no mistakes, for her tests were checked, her symptoms were getting worse, and according to her doctors it was only a matter of months before she would die. Niro decided to see things differently. By utilising the power of her spirit and following a programme very similar to what I was starting to develop for myself, she not only survived, but a year later tested HIV negative. According to conventional "wisdom" this was totally impossible. I was pretty shocked. If someone could rid their body of HIV, then I told myself that ME must be a piece of cake. Especially as there are no time constraints, such as death!

The story of Brandon Bays was equally extraordinary. In six weeks she completely healed herself of a cancerous tumour the size of a basketball. She, like Niro, achieved this by devising her own programme of healing and experiencing a remarkable psychological/spiritual transformation. The doctors once again could not explain what had happened, claiming that it must have been a miracle. In many ways it was. Amongst other things the Oxford dictionary described a miracle as "an outstanding example or achievement." I figured that this was probably rather different to the definition Brandon's doctors were referring to.

In reading about such transformations, I started to become obsessed with the notion of what creates human destiny. I continually questioned; why do some people recover from illness and not others? Why do some people live happy lives, and others just wallow in a life of pain and depression? I was beginning to realise a universal answer to these questions. The people that defy the odds in life, be that by surviving a life-threatening illness or anything else, make very different decisions. They direct their lives by setting a course and following it.

For a while I bought into the idea that people who live extraordinary lives, although they clearly do take specific actions, are simply of a different breed and are somehow stronger people with more resources. I told myself that if they were to live in my position then they would also be trapped; they, too, would see no way out. However, I soon began to realise what an easy stance this was to take. If I lived my life with that belief, then would I not just be living a self-fulfilling prophecy? Would it not mean that I would simply take the weak option when faced with a challenge, and thus live a weak life? What if I was to believe that the difference that shapes our destiny is actually the actions we take? What if I was to take those actions? Would that not also determine my destiny? Applied to ME, this simple change in my thinking translated as follows: I went from believing that it was impossible to recover from ME, to believing that it was possible. Even more importantly, I started to believe that it was not just possible for someone, but that it was actually possible for me.

My doctors might have had more training than I did in the ways of the human body, but, as I was starting to learn, that was only worth so much. Anyway, I had something they didn't: an insatiable curiosity and openness to new ideas. I wasn't going to discard something simply because conventional "wisdom" couldn't yet explain it.

However weird things often sounded, I was still willing to experiment with them on my favourite subject, me. Within these diverse parameters of course conventional medicine did also fall, and so when I did need to learn something about human anatomy and physiology I dragged my weak body off to the local library and studied until I understood what I needed to.

As I continued my research, I became fascinated by the relationship between the mind and body. Louise Hay, a prominent author in the field, had a particular impact on me. She basically worked with the philosophy that physical illness is the manifestation of dysfunctional psychological patterns. I could not fundamentally flaw her ideas. After all, this was a woman who had cured herself of terminal cancer. However, despite agreeing with the logic of her theories, and also seeing the practical implications for others, I could not see how they could benefit me. Fatigue and dizziness (still my two main symptoms) were suggested to be due to a lack of love for what one does. Yet, I was the happiest I had ever been in my life when I became ill. Sure, I hated my life now, but that was because I was ill. I started to become rather annoyed. I knew that she was right in many ways, but how could I ever have passion for life when I felt so ill? I convinced myself that my case must be different. I was very close, yet still so very far.

Autobiographies by people such as Christopher Reeve (star of the original Superman films) also provided me with much needed wisdom. For all his life Christopher Reeve had lived an existence built around his physical strength and stamina. Apart from the clear athletic needs of his work, sport was also his main source of relaxation and the place that he went for inner peace (this sounded rather familiar). One day while he was riding, he fell off his horse, with the result of being paralysed from the neck down. Totally unable to move anything but his head, for a long while his life hung in the balance. There were many times when it would have been so easy for him to die a quick natural death, as certain members of his family wished. Yet, despite the horrific events that he had been through, the frustration that he was facing everyday due to his paralysis, and the supposed hopelessness of his situation, he still had the courage to make the decision to be happy. That one decision to focus on what he had and not what he didn't, rather than the fact that once he could move and now he could not, had saved his life in more ways than one.

If Christopher Reeve could be happy, despite being able to move nothing but his head, then I knew I had nothing to complain about.

Any challenge I could ever face would be nothing in comparison. Although I did forget this many times and begin to wallow in self-pity, as soon as I reminded myself of how lucky I really was, I felt differently immediately. I was powerfully learning one of life's most important lessons:

It is not the events of our life that determine our happiness; it is the way that we respond to them.

I developed the idea that two people could go on a roller coaster, and one be screaming with joy and the other with terror. Their experience would be decided by one thing: their internal representation of the event. The person screaming with joy would be linking pleasure to the sensations in their body, and the person screaming with terror, linking fear. The physiological processes would actually be surprisingly similar. I knew which experience I wanted.

In discovering how much we really are the gatekeepers to our own happiness, I also realised the same to be true for ME, as anything else in life; if I viewed it as a living hell, then so be it, my interpretation would equal my experience. However, if I chose to view it as an adventure and an opportunity to grow into the person that I truly am, then it could equally become this.

As I slowly integrated my new understandings, a further desire started to brew in my mind. I wanted to know how I could help everyone around me to change their lives, especially my family. On numerous occasions I tried to convince them to embark on a similar journey to mine. Let's just say my ideas were not met with much support! Although the pessimism and cynicism of my environment never dampened my determination long-term, it frustrated me desperately to watch those I loved continue to destroy themselves and each other when I believed that things could be so different. I just could not understand why I could not make people change.

The gulf between my peers and myself was also becoming greater and greater. The more I searched within during my meditations and long periods of contemplation, the more I yearned to live as my true self. Yet, the qualities that I was finding to be who I really am were so different from what was seen as acceptable. I was supposed to be interested in alcohol, nightclubs and one-night stands, yet my heart was drawing me towards even more self-discovery, actualising my potential and making the world a better place. It was almost like I developed two sides to my personality. There was Alex who was still trying to be the person he believed others wanted him to be, and Alex, my spirit, who was moving towards a higher purpose. With part of me still desperate to be accepted by others, how was I now to present myself to the world? How could I explain to those around me what I was learning and discovering? I just didn't know how to interact with the world anymore. Photographs of me during this period spoke volumes, portraying a sense of "lights on, but no one home." My only reason left to live was my search for answers, and that was taking every ounce of my drained energy.

With my new passion for reading, some rather more profound questions than I had originally been asking also started to develop in my mind. Like everyone, I had always wondered, "What happens when we die?" "Are we just our bodies?" "Is there a meaning to life?" Although no one appeared to have the whole truth, some of what I was starting to read was becoming very compelling. It certainly spoke to my heart in a way that my Christian teachers hadn't. Growing up, I had attended church more than anyone else in my family, and each summer I had also gone on an adventure holiday organised by a Christian organisation. Even back then I guess I had a curiosity for answers.

I remember distinctly one summer sitting in a basement room of a beautiful school building, near to the banks of Lake Windermere in the Lake District. The school and its facilities had been hired out for a week, consisting of outdoor pursuits and games by day, and bible study and worship in the evenings. It was a tame way of being taught the Christian ways and I know that I usually enjoyed the holidays, when I wasn't being bullied anyway.

On this cool summer evening we were discussing salvation and how a person earns a place in heaven. I couldn't believe what I was hearing; it was so in contrast to what my heart was telling me Jesus had really meant. The core of the message was that if you are not a committed Christian, then you will go to hell, and even if you are a committed Christian you could still do so if you break the rules. I just could not understand how a god who created us could wish to make us suffer eternally.

"What if someone is brought up in a Muslim family?" I questioned. "What if they have never heard of Christianity?"

"Then it is for the Father to judge them," I was told. The Father of mankind judge? It made no sense to me.

"How about if someone is brought up in a Christian family, but the parents are abusive and violent and all that person sees of Christianity

69

is pain? If that persons decides to be an atheist as a consequence, would they still go to hell?" I ventured, still lost at what seemed such a ridiculous concept.

"Again, it would of course lie with God," I was told. "But without practising faith, there is little hope."

I hadn't understood at thirteen, and I still didn't five years later. Our environment creates our religious beliefs, like nearly all our beliefs. Who chooses our environment? According to Christianity, God! And, how about the fact that God is all-loving and all-powerful? If he is all-loving, then how could he condemn us? I reasoned that an all-powerful being would also be unlikely to have an ego that needs worshipping! Unfortunately, this was not to be my last run in with such illogical thinking.

I knew that many Christians live amazing lives, growing themselves and helping others; it was neither they nor their faith that I had a problem with. It was those who take religious understandings and twist them into a way of controlling people that frustrated me. I reasoned that it must surely be the highest arrogance to believe you are better than other people because you hold a certain set of beliefs. To me, this was at about the same level as football hooliganism: fighting someone because they are wearing a different T-shirt.

My understanding was that many people have an experience of "God," and then assume that only those of their faith could be having such experiences "legitimately." Any spiritual experience outside that religion is therefore condemned and claimed to be the result of the devil or evil spirits. I gave up trying to reason with such beliefs. If you yourself hold such dogmatic beliefs, I have no wish to convert you to the devil's ways; this is a book about how I changed my life, not about consorting with the dark side. Please read on, and do not be put off that we see the world differently. In the spirit of my favourite comedian, and the great Scottish philosopher, Billy Connolly: I'm the one going to hell; you are just reading about it!

Thursday nights at the meditation group were becoming more and more fascinating, and less and less tame. Channelling was something that after a few months we started experimenting with. I was, at first, again highly sceptical. I was also rather fearful. The idea that it is possible to contact the dead, and that there are "higher" spiritual entities in existence, also meant that there is more guiding our lives than just us. Although other people in the group would "get stuff through," I was pretty useless and never got anything (my being too terrified to relax probably contributed to this). However, one visit to a professional and I knew that, when done properly, there is clearly more than guesswork involved.

The channel I saw was Edwin Courtenay (quite famous in certain circles). As I walked out of the appointment, I did what I am sure many people do, I tried to conceive of a way in which he could have produced the information that he did through less ethical means. I immediately discounted the use of body language, for Edwin had had his eyes closed throughout, and the information was far too specific to have been read from non-verbal cues anyway. For a moment I considered that it might have been possible for him to research my life before he saw me, but there was no way he could have done this without my awareness. There was also the reality that he was working full-time and could not possibly research everyone that he saw. After listening to the tape of the session several times, there was only one conclusion I could draw: channelling was for real.

Apart from explaining the dynamics of a number of family relationships with incredible accuracy, Edwin essentially confirmed what I was already starting to believe, that I had chosen my illness before I was born as a way to wake me up to my true self. I was also told that I had lived many past lives in close contact to famous teachers such as Merlin and St. Germain. Apparently in one of my incarnations I was attuned to the "Violet Flame," an extremely powerful healing energy used to create dramatic transformations in peoples' lives. Although quietly chuffed at being told that I was "special," I figured that everyone has similar experiences. Upon playing the tape to Shirley, my meditation teacher, I was told in no uncertain terms that this was not the case. This did no end of magic for my seriously confused self-image.

However, despite being convinced that Edwin was for real, I was still on the whole sceptical about mediums and channels. It seemed to me that even if someone is in contact with an entity it does not mean that his or her perceptions are the whole, or even partial, truth; for someone to channel, the information has to come through his or her own personality. In addition, I reasoned that being dead or from other places is hardly an automatic boost to genius level. After all, people have committed suicide acting on channelled information. I figured that in many ways, great channelling is like using a water filter: you need relatively clean water (information) in the first place, as well as a good quality filter (channel).

71

Probably the most inspiring example of channelling that I found was a series of books by Neale Donald Walsch, entitled "Conversations with God." Once again I had unearthed another extraordinary story of personal transformation. It all began when one day Neale sat down and wrote a letter to God, explaining his grievances and frustrations with life. Many people have done such things, and for them that has been the end of the story; they eventually pull themselves together and get on with their life much as before. However, in the case of Neale it was different. As soon as he stopped writing his letter, the pen continued to move. God was writing an answer!

Over the next few years, Neale channelled a total of three books: the first covering personal truths, the second global truths, and the third the really big questions. The books made for remarkable reading, and answered many questions I had about religion and spirituality in a way that was both simple and logical. Things that have been the subject of wars and conflicts of so many kinds, were dealt with in a way which just gave me that "Oh yeah, I can't believe I never got this!" feeling.

Reading books such as these, as well as ancient teachings from various Eastern religions, assisted me in developing my own sense of God and spirituality. I started to realise that all the great religions agree on the fundamentals, essentially that there is more to life than there appears and that we should love one another while being true to ourselves. Although not wishing to join any particular religion, such a sense of faith in life and the universe became invaluable to me.

As my understanding deepened, I also started to notice a larger force working in my life. Countless small coincidences started to happen, such as developing a question in my mind, only to find the answer in the next chapter of a book I was reading. Little did I know it at the time, but the more we are open to such guidance the more powerful it gets. Thank God this is the case, for it would not be long before I would desperately need such wisdom.

CHAPTER 12: THINGS HEAT UP (SPRING 1999)

I guess it comes down to a simple choice really: get busy living or
get busy dying.
The Shawshank Redemption

Being on my healing programme for six months, the benefits were starting to become noticeable. I was already sleeping on average two hours less a day, and I was feeling more focused than I could ever remember being. Yet despite this, I still felt ill the whole time and was still struggling with even the lightest of exercise. Even attempting to increase my yoga and qigong to more than ten minutes a day was taking serious effort and, apart from developing the mental muscle of perseverance, I wondered what good such a short period of time could actually be doing? However, I kept at it, telling myself that the most important thing was that I was getting the blood and energy in my body moving.

As I continued to work on myself, I realised that an undeniable psychological shift was starting to take place. I was beginning to believe that my illness might in fact have been the best thing to have ever happened to me, for it was leading me to insights I might have never otherwise had. It was also giving me a unique opportunity to consider the insanity of the world around me. The standard day of most people I knew was to need coffee (effectively a drug) to get out of bed in the morning, to spend eight hours doing something pointless and boring, to return home and fail to relate to their loved ones, before using another drug (i.e. alcohol, food or television) to numb the pain and assist in falling asleep again, only to get up the next day and repeat the cycle. The price of several years of illness to learn how to avoid such an existence seemed almost reasonable.

With my new lifestyle permeating every corner of my life, my schoolwork did not remain untouched. My teachers had gone from suggesting that I leave school because I was so far behind, to reluctantly basing my exam predictions on the pieces of work that I had been able to complete, meaning I was predicted a highly respectable three B's. This change had taken only six months. However, I wasn't satisfied. Having read several books on human potential and self-belief, I decided to set a higher standard. Knowing I needed a goal which would drive me, I decided to aim for three A's, something that was almost unheard of. The idea of defying the odds, not only with my recovery, but also with the rest of my life, was exciting me more and more.

Around this time I began to become interested in the phenomena known as energy healing, in part spurred on by reading about the experiences of Iain's wife, Renate, described in his book "Close Encounters." Before her awakening, Renate was happily married with two children and living an idyllic life as a housewife in Vienna. One day she started to have spiritual experiences, such as spontaneously leaving her body for no apparent reason. Before she knew it, her whole life was like a tornado, gathering more and more energy. She was being pulled towards an uncertain future and a way of life that could not have been further away from the security that until this point she had known. Thankfully for the hundreds of people whom she had helped since these experiences, she was courageous enough to trust the process of life and follow the invisible path that was being laid down for her. Ever since that time, she had lived all over the world and used her gift to heal people.

Another incredible healing story I came across was that of Gene Egidio. In one week his entire life fell apart. On the Monday his marriage of twenty-five years finally ended in the divorce courts. On the Tuesday his business partner absconded with all the company's funds. On the Wednesday he had a dramatic head-on car accident where he broke several ribs and wrote off his car. On the Thursday he lost his legal rights to two other companies in which he was financially involved, and on the Friday someone stole all his business equipment. Over the next few months he lost all his savings, along with various properties he owned, and was finally declared bankrupt, even reaching the point of having to sell his watch for food money.

Three months after Gene's week from hell, a lady he hardly knew called him up on the telephone and explained she had dreamed of him healing her of a sickness she had. She pushed him to let her come to his house, and, unable to find a way to say "no," Gene reluctantly agreed. When the lady arrived, she was covered from head to toe in blisters and he discovered she was suffering from herpes. You can imagine what went through his head: "What next, herpes?" After introducing herself, she sat down, took his hands and put them on her shoulders. A few minutes later, somewhat embarrassed, he tried to pull them away. He couldn't; they were stuck. Gene thought he had gone mad and seriously started to question his own sanity.

After around thirty minutes Gene's hands finally became free and the lady got up and left. The next day she called in a hysterical state. She had been totally cured! There was not a single mark on her body.

After she had been to the doctor and come round to show Gene for himself, he sat down feeling rather bemused and fell asleep. He woke up three days later.

As Gene awoke, he felt as though his whole body was being filled with energy, to the point that it was overflowing out of his head. He also started experiencing incredible sensations of feeling the energy in everything and everyone. He could actually sense the connection that exists between all matter. He got up, walked to the front door and left his house, never to return. Ever since then healing had been his calling. Some of the cases he cited in his book were just extraordinary, including cases of people being permanently healed of terminal illnesses in a matter of minutes. To me this was absolutely mind-blowing, and also totally fascinating. What if I could be healed of ME, was the obvious question that was starting to brew in my strengthening mind.

In researching quantum physics and the science behind healing, I discovered that atoms and particles, what scientists had thought to be the smallest elements, are actually made of pure energy. In essence this meant that energy is the building block of everything that exists. The writings of Deepak Chopra impacted me especially. A highly respected endocrinologist, he explained how the cells in our body are constantly regenerating; for example we have a new liver every six weeks, new skin every three to four weeks, a new stomach lining every four days, and new eyes every two days! In fact, ninety-eight percent of the cells in our body are replaced every year. This meant that the body I had had over two years ago when I had originally got ill didn't even exist anymore. This being the case, I questioned why I was still ill. Deepak Chopra's argument was that inside of our cells are "phantom memories" which maintain our illness, and that those who experience remarkable healing are tapping into these "phantom memories" and changing them. It seemed to me that using healing energy would be a powerful way to do this.

In considering the history of healing, I thought about how many people claim to believe in the miracles that Jesus performed, but doubt that such things are still possible. I questioned how this could be the case. After all, the structure of the world has not changed in the last two thousand years. The reality appeared to me to be more that people have been conditioned to take a pill instead. I was sure that the vast profits made by drug manufacturers were just a coincidence and played no role in this!

Studies conducted with one of the most famous healers in Britain, Mathew Manning, provided me with further indisputable evidence in support of healing. Scientists had found him able to take seeds in his hands, and in a matter of minutes make them sprout and grow several inches. Faith played no part, unless of course seeds hold beliefs?

One Thursday night at the meditation group there was talk of Reiki, a form of healing that anyone can learn. For the price of £30 (incredibly cheap compared to the hundreds of pounds many people pay) a local woman was attuning people. Being drawn along by the energy of the group, I decided to sign up. I have to admit that, as with most things, I went along needing to be convinced. I reasoned that healing is a gift you either have or you don't have, rather like song writing or painting. I wasn't really sure that it was something you could be attuned to. What I was to discover is that although there are those who are gifted, it is also possible to learn healing, just as it is possible to learn how to write a song or to paint. There are the Phil Collins' and Bob Dylan's, and the Michelangelo's and Picasso's, and then there are also those that can still do great works, despite never reaching the level of the masters. As I had learnt song writing, I was also to learn healing.

The first time that I connected with Reiki energy was pretty powerful. Some people feel the energy as a heat, others as a tingling or vibration. As far as I was concerned it felt like all three! For almost every day after my attunements, I was to use the energy with myself, often for as much as an hour at a time.

Like other things I had experienced over the previous months, most people I knew dismissed Reiki and healing as rubbish and a sure sign that my years of illness were further taking their toll on my sanity. But, if anyone really was interested in intelligent discussion, I did have a rather compelling argument. I would point out that for many years the only evidence supporting the idea of radio waves was that you could hear them, and that the only difference with healing energy is that it is a feeling rather than a sound. I also explained that the man who invented the radio was nearly put in a mental institution when he talked of his idea. People just could not conceive of it as being possible, and only after experiencing it for themselves did they go from being disbelieving to being amazed. I would finally question anyone who would listen, that, with one in two people in the Western world dying from heart disease, and one in three dying from cancer, can we honestly believe that traditional medicine holds all the answers?

My attunements to Reiki, along with my many hours spent in

meditation, started to have a rather profound effect on my energy system. I remember on one occasion waking up in the middle of the night and my whole body vibrating with energy, to the point that I could even hear it. For a few moments I felt my old feelings of anxiety rising, but I soon settled myself by focusing on the potential positives, praying that I might wake up the next morning dramatically healed. Although upon waking I was to be disappointed, the experience did give me a sense of encouragement, along with an even stronger belief in the power of what I was doing. On numerous occasions whilst I was meditating I also had various strange visions and sensations in my body. After a while I just took them as par for the course as well.

However, despite the clear transformation of my internal world, my physical health was still only improving at a painfully slow rate. There were many times that my progress was so minute that I could barely see it. In fact, often the only way to notice even a slight improvement was to look back on how I had been several months previously. Thankfully, my lack of other options saved me from giving up. In addition, I used a very scary question to keep myself focused; what were the chances of someone developing a universal cure for ME that was even 50% effective in the next ten years? I reasoned that I wouldn't back a horse on those odds. Why then had I backed that same horse with the last two years of my life?

I would also repeat in my head a quote by a famous marathon runner:

It doesn't matter how many times you give up along the way, as long as you keep putting one foot in front of the other.

I remember one Sunday evening around this time escaping from the hustle and bustle of a family birthday in an upstairs bedroom at my grandparents. Iain and Renate were sitting with me for a while whilst I rested. They had been a regular source of focus over the past months and tonight was no different.

"Still no magic pill," I said half jokingly, with a look of defeat creeping onto my face. It was meant as a joke, but it held too much truth to really be funny.

"Well, there is a magic pill," Iain replied, "But it is nothing on the outside. In essence, it is a magic pill within. It is the power you use to change your life and find your own answers. It is your own determination and commitment to create a way when the environment around you suggests that there isn't one."

I knew Iain was right, and I was still slowly healing, for the time being anyway.

By Easter my progress was finally becoming more obviously noticeable. I was now only sleeping for twenty minutes in the afternoon and under ten hours at night. Although I was still lying around most of the day resting and reading, this was a major improvement from the past two years. Since starting my programme I had cut my sleep by about three hours a day, and that meant an extra three hours a day to spend searching for my cure.

My schoolwork was also starting to come together. For the final three months before exams, I reasoned I had an average of about four hours a day that I could effectively study. That meant I basically had three hundred hours to teach myself a significant portion of two years' work. Compared to the challenge of curing myself from severe ME it seemed pretty straightforward! I drew up a detailed timetable and broke each day up into three time slots with intermittent rest breaks. Using the same determination and dedication that I was using to slowly transform my health, I got to work.

With the now real possibility of passing my A-levels, it was also necessary to make some decisions regarding my future. Before my illness I had guessed that if my ambitions to be a musician did not work out I would probably go to university, read something like business studies or economics, and then one day get a job in London. However, things were now different. Perhaps in part because of my desperate need to understand my family and myself, the books that I had been reading on psychology spoke to me in a way I had never known before. In many ways it was like I was reminding myself of wisdom I already knew, rather than reading such books for the first time. I figured that going to university would be a great way to further develop my newly realised passion, whilst at the same time continuing my journey of healing. Even more importantly than that, university would also offer the chance of a new life away from the constant hell that I had been sharing with those I loved.

With my teachers' reluctant prediction of three B's, I could go pretty much wherever I wanted. There were a few restrictions though: accommodation in London would be too expensive, and a university more than a couple of hours drive away would be difficult for my family to get to (something that suited me just fine). But, regardless of any of this, I really had only one criterion – I had to be by the sea. I didn't know why, for I had never even lived nearer than an hours drive from the coast. Yet, I had spent enough time over the past six months listening to my heart to know what it was asking for, and living by the sea was it. I therefore sat down with Mum and we went through all the seaside towns that had universities. Included in these were Southampton, Brighton, and Bournemouth, but none of them sounded right. Then, on the off chance, Mum said Swansea, although immediately dismissed it, saying it was too far away and her mind drifted towards other nearer universities.

Something strange happened to me all of a sudden. It may sound like another sign of my insanity, but I knew, without any doubt, that Swansea was the place where my recovery could continue. I had not seen a prospectus, I knew nothing about the university's reputation, and I had never even been there. But none of this mattered, I still knew. From that moment on it was only a matter of convincing everyone else that it was the right place for me, despite it being half a day's drive away and not at the top of the league tables (although I was later to discover that it did have one of the best psychology departments in Europe). With my new grasp of psychology and what motivates people's choices in life, this was actually surprisingly easy!

As I started back at school for my last term I was feeling very confident. As far as I was concerned I was going to achieve grades higher than anyone would be able to believe, I was going to continue to regain my health and, after the summer, I would be living in another country studying what I was passionate about. I could not conceive of anything that could stop me. That was, apart from ME.

CHAPTER 13: THE FIRE EXTINGUISHES – MY DARKEST DAYS (SUMMER 1999)

In the depth of Winter, I finally learned that within me there lay an invincible Summer.
Albert Camus

After a few weeks back at school, I was still feeling confident and enjoying the intellectually superior position that the past two months of focused study had earned me. No one I spoke to had done anything like the amount of work I had, despite the comparable ease of their situations. It felt so good to actually be ahead, after having spent the last three years desperately trying to catch up. It also did wonders for my self-belief to have turned my studies around so dramatically in such a short period of time.

Three weeks before my first exam, I took a night off to go and see one of my favourite bands of all time, Silverchair. I had been too ill to go to gigs until now, except for those that I had played in, and prior to the night I was incredibly excited that a little dream was coming true. However, the event actually turned out to be rather depressing; it simply reminded me how alien I now was from a world I had once loved.

Silverchair were a hard rock band, and consequently attracted the "alternative" music crowd. Hundreds of people singing along to songs about how terrible life is and how we are all victims of a condemned society no longer inspired me. For the first time I was actually relieved that Sugarkane had never gone places. However lonely my new path was becoming, at least it was leading somewhere different. My future simply did not lie around people focusing their lives on pain and depression.

Crawling into bed that night and feeling the comfort of my sheets hold me once again was a major relief. Yet my sleep was not restful. I simply could not relax. Despite my incredible exhaustion, my mind just would not slow down. After many hours of frustration, I eventually drifted off around 5:00 and so awoke the next morning feeling completely wiped out. I had overdone it and knew I was going to have to pay the price for a couple of days. At the same time, I had been studying intensely and I figured it would do me good to slow down for a while before I had to turn the intensity up even further for my final exams.

By the middle of the next week there was still nothing to suggest that this time was any different to other occasions when I had done too

80

much. I was starting to feel better, and although it was a struggle, I managed to take a three-hour mock history exam on the Wednesday afternoon. The room had been spinning for most of the time, but this was something I was used to by now.

But, as I tried to relax into the bath the evening after the exam, my body started to re-enter some old territory that I thought I had left behind. The intensity of my dizziness from the day started to rapidly multiply. What had been a quiet uneasy tune playing in the background was once again becoming an in-your-face rock anthem, just like when I had struggled on stage with Sugarkane. I once again felt like someone else was in control of my mind and body.

As I tried to rest in the water and ignore what was happening inside me, it felt like the room was starting to shake. Suddenly losing consciousness, I grasped at the sides of the bath. A second or two later I came round and tried to take a deep breath. It was no good; it started happening again. My heart began to pump blood at an award-winning rate. I attempted to fight it. I forced myself to lie down and struggled to relax; hoping that whatever it was would leave me alone. The day was over now, surely if there was anything wrong it would have already got me, I tried to reason. It wasn't working. I was feeling worse and worse. I started to pass out again. My terror hit the roof.

There was no one else in the house. I might lose consciousness properly and drown, I tortured myself. I would not be found for hours. I had to get out of the bath. I had to get help. I really needed someone around, someone to save me from the hell I could feel brewing inside. As quickly as I could, I dragged myself out of the water and stumbled across the landing into my mum's bedroom to get to the telephone, bumping into pretty much every wall on the way. After a number of attempts, I managed to dial my grandmother's house, where Mum was visiting for the evening. As the telephone began to ring, for a few moments I started to feel pathetic for needing to call for help at my age, but a second later the terror swept me up again and all I could feel was my out-of-control fear. My reality was that I needed someone around. In no uncertain terms I told Mum to get back as quickly as possible.

Mum came rushing through the door fifteen minutes later to find me sitting on the sofa shaking, trying to distract my mind by watching television. Although I was able to focus my eyes again, I was still totally and utterly terrified. What had just happened? Why had it happened? I thought I had done everything right to get better. I had read dozens of books and religiously stuck to my meditation and other practices. I had also visited everyone I could find; I was even currently under a new homeopath that had cured over a hundred people with identical symptoms to mine. Why was nothing working? Why was I still so ill?

It was not until I had recovered from the immediate terror of that night that I really started to enter the darkest period of my life. Although it was certainly not the first time things had collapsed around me, this time I didn't have the time or motivation to rebuild them. After committing every spare moment of nine months of my life to changing everything about myself I could, I was once again back where I had started. It felt like there was nothing left to try. I couldn't have worked any harder than I had. I had continually stuck to my healing programme, even through times when I had desperately wanted just to curl up and watch television. There had been numerous occasions when the last thing I wanted was to read another book about other people's lives changing, yet I had still kept on going.

Why? I kept asking. Why was this happening to me? Why me? Even my desire to defy the medical institution had now gone. What was the point anyway? All that "change your life" bullshit was a waste of fucking time, it had just been more false hope, more lies, and more of my life wasted, my disillusionment continued.

I once again spent my existence just lying in front of the television for days on end, trying to numb my mind and escape the world. It no longer worked. Even that retreat had been taken from me. Every day that my exams got a step closer, I got a step closer to my final chance of freedom being stolen. All those hours pushing through a spinning room to try to keep up with the mountains of essays towering all around me, all those hours I forced myself to go to school when I could hardly walk, would they all really count for nothing? I couldn't even sit in a chair for more than about five minutes without starting to pass out. How would I be able to write even one essay in this state, let alone the sixteen my exams required?

The almost certain loss of my escape to Swansea added further to my torture. The new friends I had dreamed of and my life by the sea, they were to have been my saving grace and key to a new life. There seemed to be no point left in anything, I may as well have spent the last nine months watching television, I reasoned. That scary question, the question that drives most people who attempt to kill themselves, was burning brighter than ever before in my desperate mind; what is the point?

By the time exams were about to start, I was just able to lie on the sofa and read through my notes for a couple of hours each day; but sitting at a desk was still absolute torture. My head would spin and my whole body would break out in a sweat, which only ceased once I returned my body to a restful horizontal position. Most of my exams were three hours long. That meant three years of absolute hell trying to survive at school were going to come down to my ability to complete three-hour exams when I could barely even sit at a desk. I just couldn't envisage how it was possible. However, I refused to give up, trying to do as much work as I conceivably could, thankful at least that I had studied so hard over recent months. But, I reasoned it wouldn't be enough; until this point I had been working on organising the information I needed to use, along with structuring my arguments. It was at this time now that I was supposed to be committing everything to memory.

One Saturday night, a few days before my first exam, is etched into my memory for eternity. My mum and stepfather had gone out for dinner and I had been left alone in the house. It was about 9:00 and I was taking my plates out to the kitchen, in the middle of watching some rubbish on television. As I walked towards the dishwasher, a knife on the kitchen surface caught my eye. Looking at it shining in front of me, a permanent answer to all my problems stared right at me. Just a few cuts and the whole thing would be over. I had at least two hours until my mum and stepfather returned. It would be more than long enough for me to escape.

With my ever-growing depression by now blackening my whole being, I could no longer see anything apart from the darkness. I continually questioned: why even fucking try? I was born; my father left. I grew up; I was never good enough. I went to school; the other kids hated me. I escaped through sport; I got ill. I loved music; it went nowhere. I had given everything to my attempted recovery; it had failed too. I had no friends, no hobbies, no love in my life, and there was no conceivable way out. I may as well end it now, I reasoned. There was actually something quite peaceful about the thought of death. To me dying just meant going back home and ending the suffering. It would be like the perfect holiday. It would be perfect because it would be permanent. It felt like swapping hell for heaven, an easy choice to make.

By this time I was too numb to scream and I was too numb to cry. I was too numb to feel anything apart from desperation and depression. I wasn't even locking my pain away anymore; there was nowhere left to put it. I lived in a fantasy world that I created moment to moment in my mind. In this world I was famous and married to a beautiful popstar, people cared about me, and my family were proud of me. I had friends and I had a reason to live. I loved my life, I loved the world, and so did everyone else.

The times that I realised I had been fantasising a dream world, reality once again struck me like a sledgehammer and I desperately craved to escape again. Fuck self-awareness, I screamed inside; I wanted to be asleep like the rest of the world. That knife would put me to rest permanently. I remembered that it had been sharpened recently; it would do a perfect job. I knew this was very different to the times in the past when my sister had tried to commit suicide. Those where cries for help. This was not going to be a cry for help. I was not willing to fail again.

So much for all of that spiritual crap I had been reading, my horrible mind ranted. Where was God now? If the universe was guiding my life, then why the fuck was I feeling this way? How about my family, where were they when I needed them? Why were they so immersed in their own shit? Why was no one ever there for me? Why did no one love me? If the answers were inside me, then why the hell had I not found them? I had been desperately searching for nine solid months and I was now even worse off. I couldn't even relate to my favourite music anymore.

The more I learnt about the human personality, the more all I could see was what a fucked up mess the world is in. Why would a world of such brutality even be created? I didn't want to be a part of it anymore. It was time to end it all. It was time to go back home. Beginning to make my decision, I breathed a sigh of relief.

As I picked up the knife it spoke to me, "You know you are ready," it said. "I'll take away the pain," it promised. "Just do what you are desperate to do," it tempted me, "End it once and for all." I felt the handle teasing my fingers. It was the perfect weight. What a way to end the darkness, I thought, with both a sinking sensation and a feeling of elation all at once. I started to imagine its sharp blade gently caressing my skin as it moved closer.

Just before I started to cut though, for one last moment I considered my options. I had to know from the bottom of my heart that I was doing the right thing. I knew that once I started I wouldn't stop. I did still have one feeling of unease: what if the universe really was guiding me? What if the problem was only that it wasn't the guidance I wanted? What if I needed to fall this low for a reason? What if this was exactly as had been planned for my life, perhaps even by me?

I began to remember all the stories of personal change that I had read. In every single case of dramatic transformation I had come across, the deepest realisations had come after times of intense searching, and often also deep suffering. Part of my mind tried to reason that they were other people's lives and that I was different. Perhaps my low was lower than their lows, it tried to convince me. Yet, something told me that such thoughts were just a cop out.

The lives of people such as Niro Markoff Asistent, Brandon Bays, Louise Hay, Christopher Reeve and Gene Egidio had only been transformed so incredibly because they had had the courage to keep on going. If they had given in when things got tough, then their stories would never have ended the way they had. Of course my mind also had a response to this: I was only eighteen years old. These people had all been at least twice my age when they had faced their demons. They had had independence, emotional support, and years more life experience. Here I was stuck at home, surrounded by depression, with nothing but my determination and faith to keep me going. With even these wavering, did I really have enough to keep fighting? I knew that I would only ever find out if I tried.

My heart retched as I put the knife down. The thought of going on made me want to be sick. I still wasn't sure that I could face what I knew was coming. There was one thing for certain: if I was going to keep going, there was no way that life could ever be the same again. My quest had to have a different meaning; recovering from ME was no longer enough to drive me through the darkness. My life came down to one final choice: I was either going to kill myself, or I was going to do whatever it took to create the life of my dreams.

It was in making this choice that I saved myself. If I had not spent the previous nine months on the voyage that I had, my decision would have been very different. If I had not believed deep down that there was an alternative and that I would find it, there is no way you would be reading these words, and I would probably be dead. Along with my faith, I did have one other saving grace: a core belief that we are here on earth for a reason. I believed that to run away could well have made things worse, for if I had done so, then I would only have had to learn my lessons another way.

In making my decision to create the life of my dreams, I felt a strange knowing inside. It was that same knowing I had had about

Swansea. Although I could barely hear it in the midst of my terrifying hopelessness, it was somehow attempting to communicate a message to me, telling me that I was not as alone as I thought I was. Not for many years would I find out who the voice was.

As it was clear there was no way I would be able to take my exams under normal conditions, alternatives were considered. It seemed that there were none. Waiting was not an option; I would probably not emotionally survive another year in my current circumstances. The headmaster of St. John's was telephoned to see if I could take the exams at home, for at least then I would have been able to cut out the twenty-minute journey to and from school. Despite Mum's pleas he refused; there seemed to be no way to communicate the intensity of the illness that I was experiencing. The only help he was willing to offer was to let me sit my papers in the sanatorium at school, meaning I could take regular rests during my papers. It felt like little consolation, for the journey to and from school each day was going to be like running a marathon before and after what was already looking like a one man Olympic games. Yet, even though I was only getting minimal support from the school, having made the decision to live, I knew that I had to face my demons. Risking making myself so ill that I ended up in hospital, psychiatric or otherwise, was better than the thought of continuing another year where I was.

The following three weeks were, without doubt, the worst of my life. Life was total and utter sheer, uncompromising, hell. I had never suffered like that before, and I had never seen anyone else go through something similar. Worse than the physical pain was the emotional torture. The hours I was awake I could barely concentrate for a minute, and I could hardly even sit straight in a chair. Writing my papers, I was at times barely even able to focus on the desk in front of me. Thinking was also immensely difficult; my brain was just an intense fog of darkness. I simply turned answering the questions over to my unconscious mind, which I hoped was saying the right things; it certainly shocked me on more than one occasion when answers just seemed to appear out of nowhere. As soon as I finished each exam I was onto the next, trying to get some minimal preparatory work done in the middle of my never-ending need for sleep.

Thankfully, winter does not last forever; spring always arrives eventually. After spring comes summer, and one day soon the sun would start to shine again in my life. I had no real way of knowing, but the universe really was still guiding me. Iain had come across another healer who he felt might be of use. His methods were to make Ravi's look conventional. His name was Jack Temple, and he was a dowser and homeopath who had gathered his own remedies from around the world. At that time, the summer of 1999, a media frenzy was riding around him, due to his treating famous people such as The Princess of Wales, The Duchess of York and Jerry Hall. He had also been featured in national papers such as "The Daily Telegraph" and "The Observer," and was about to star in a BBC television documentary.

The bizarre thing was that I got the last available appointment as a new patient before the television show jammed the appointment book and waiting list (which closed at 1,000 people); it was the day after my last exam, the first appointment in the morning. This was the first consultation that I could conceivably have made. Maybe this was just a coincidence, but I chose to believe it was not. Even if there was no benefit, it didn't matter; it gave me hope. It was this hope that just pulled me through. Going through hell was always going to be tough, but it was a darn sight easier at the times I felt I had something guiding me. My faith that had almost totally disappeared was starting to rekindle.

CHAPTER 14: DO OR DIE - MY LAST CHANCE

When written in Chinese, the word crisis is composed of two characters.
One represents danger and the other represents opportunity.
John F. Kennedy

Sitting in Jack Temple's office the first morning after my exams was an incredible relief. I just hoped that I had done enough to achieve the grades I needed to get to Swansea. Just to think of not escaping from the world around me was itself terrifying. Watching Jack work on me, I was reminded of the same wonder I had experienced in the presence of Ravi. Here was another person who really knew what he was talking about; Jack Temple was over eighty years old, needed only a few hours' sleep, exercised every day, and was re-growing the hair on his head.

For nearly half an hour I sat there in a mixture of awe and amusement as Jack asked his pendulum questions and scribbled down pieces of information. To think of the supposedly amazing advances of modern medicine, and I had more faith in an old-age pensioner holding a crystal on the end of a piece of string! Looking around the office, three of the walls were covered from floor to ceiling in bottles containing remedies, much like the cave of a medieval alchemist. Many of them Jack had himself collected from distant locations all over the world.

After a while, Jack got out about three or four remedies, stuck them to some masking tape, and then taped them to my arms. He told me that I had certain poisons in my body blocking the flow of my energy and I was to leave the patches on for a couple of hours to draw them out. He could see no reason why I would not make a full recovery by the time I was due to leave for Wales.

Although seriously impressed by Jack's display of his obvious abilities, my cynicism, developed over three years of being let down, questioned, how was this time going to be any different to other occasions I had seen medical gurus. What could Jack have that the others hadn't? Yet, by the time I left, my cynicism had already given way to my ever-eternal optimism. Of course it would work, I convinced myself. I spent the journey home feeling as confident as ever I had found my magic pill.

After several more appointments I was rather less hopeful. Although I had slowly recovered to the level of health that I had been at before my exams, Jack seemed unable to take me beyond it. I was starting to realise that for some reason my case was not like others. I was now baffling the complementary health experts, just as I had the doctors. Thankfully, I was no longer asking the "Why?" questions, I just once again got back to my internal search.

Something that started to enter my mind was that I needed to have more fun. My life seemed to be a constant effort, for even now, when I was supposed to be on holiday, all I ever did was continually focus on my recovery. With every spare moment I was reading the latest nutritional theory or another ancient teaching on the meaning of life. While once again doing my daily commitments, in an attempt to get a social life I started trying to go out with my old music friends, who were back from university for the summer. It was worse than I imagined. We had nothing left in common. Their world no longer made any sense to me. The only way I could come close to being accepted was to pretend to be something I was not, and even then I wasn't fooling anyone, least of all myself. At times, the loneliness felt almost unbearable. Yet, somehow I managed to use my confused self-image as a catalyst to drive my inner searching even harder.

After spending a few days staying with my uncle, I was guided to realise the potential benefits of gentle walking. Because walking was something that rapidly drained the little energy I had, until this point I had avoided using my muscles as much as possible. However, the consequent result was that my body had almost totally wasted away, and I was now extremely underweight. In an attempt to slowly rectify my severe de-conditioning, I started walking for twenty minutes each day. Just this took much of my newfound determination, along with a very steady mind to counteract my still severe dizziness. But, by the end of the summer, I was gradually becoming stronger and able to walk slowly for twenty-five minutes a day. I just hoped that my energy was reaching a place where I would be able to look after myself at university, assuming of course I had passed my exams.

The morning of my results I telephoned my tutor to hear my fate, knowing that the last year of my unbeatable commitment to creating my own cure, of the sort of determination it takes to climb a mountain like Everest, was all going to come down to this. My future was about to be decided. Had I managed three B's? No, I hadn't. I had failed to meet the requirements set for me by the school. I had lived to my own standards instead. I had straight A's. I was top of the school, and had also won the award for business studies and tied for the economics award.

How I managed to score the incredible grades I did under such circumstances is something that blew away a lot of people. My family were ecstatic and my teachers seriously confused. Despite my immense personal relief, my celebrations were bittersweet. I would have traded my exam results for full health without a second thought.

The rest of the summer passed quickly, and at last it was time to leave my past behind. After what had felt like an eternity, I was going to leave my prison of pain and isolation. It was time to move to Wales. For the first time in as long as I could remember I was actually excited, really excited, about life. I had made it. I had found my way out. I was about to enter a new world. What did it have in store for me?

CHAPTER 15: REBIRTH (AUTUMN 1999 TO SUMMER 2000)

Out of every crisis comes the chance to be reborn, to reconceive ourselves as individuals, to choose the kind of change that will help us to grow and to fulfil ourselves more completely.
Nena O'Neill

As the car pulled away and I said goodbye to my family, I looked back at the house I had lived in since I was seven, the place where for the last three years I had spent almost my entire existence in one state: the state of illness. On our route to the motorway, Mum and I passed both my secondary school and St. John's, with the countryside in between attempting to deceive me into a sense of nostalgia. I felt no sorrow at leaving, and not an ounce of fear at the massive changes that lay ahead; I was just consumed by total and utter relief at having a new start. No longer would I have to be the victim of the pains of those I loved.

As we reached the monotonous and boring M4, a powerful feeling of destiny was burning in me. Although I wasn't naïve enough anymore to think that everything in my life would now be perfect, my heart was telling me that I was finally in for a break, along with an opportunity to gain some perspective. When we are locked in our life, be it painful or pleasurable, we tend to think that everyone is living the same way. It is scientifically proven that people in a happy state remember a much higher percentage of happy incidents, and that people in a negative state remember a higher percentage of negative ones. Well, I certainly connected with the second of these. Hell was not an abstract concept for me; it had been my home for much of my life.

Seeing the waves rolling onto the golden sands of Swansea bay that first afternoon, it struck me even more powerfully how incredible the guidance in our lives is. I just prayed that those I was leaving behind would one day be able to listen to similar wisdom. But, by now I had learnt to leave their transformation to the universe. If it were meant to be, then I would be there in a second to help.

As I settled into university life, it felt fantastic to be meeting so many diverse and interesting people. No longer wearing the masks I had in the past, I found myself able to relate to others in a whole new way. Ever since I had been bullied at primary and secondary school, I had always been concerned with being accepted by the "cool" crowd and trying to be popular, even if I didn't feel it. I now looked for different qualities in people. I was far less concerned with being around people who wore the "right" label clothes, listened to the "right" bands, or said the "right" things at the "right" times. I was now drawn to people for who they were in terms of their ability to communicate their own humanness and spirit.

With much of my passion for life regained, I even became involved in student radio, meaning that for two hours a week I had my own radio show, where I played an assortment of pop and rock music and chatted about various topics of interest. Having been a spectator of society for so long it felt fantastic to once again participate.

By the end of the first semester I was still thriving. It was such a relief to know that I was managing to look after myself, even with my still very limited energy. Unfortunately, I was still spending many hours of the day severely fatigued and, however hard I tried, I just could not stay awake in the afternoons. Yet, my determination never wavered; full health was still an obsession, even in the middle of my new life.

In my constant search to find ways to accelerate my healing, one of the realisations I had was of the importance of developing my fitness. I therefore took yoga and walking, the two forms of exercise that I knew were within my capability, and made increasing my tolerance to them a priority. I figured that the time of day when I would feel most like exercising, and also when I would be the least likely to get distracted, was first thing in the morning. Consequently, for five mornings a week of my second semester, I dragged myself out of bed at what felt like the crack of dawn to exercise. It excited me so much to know that I was now in a position where I could do this, with the only price being my needing extra sleep in the afternoon. By the end of the second term I was power walking (running was still out of the question) for forty minutes every morning, that was after I had completed my twenty minutes' yoga. Although my new friends were often awed at my incredible discipline, only I knew what it had really taken to get myself this far.

Some of my best experiences that first year involved storming along the golden sands, flying past the dog walkers and watching the sun climbing above Swansea bay. It was my sanctuary away from the busy life of the university campus where I lived. It was also where for the first time in years I felt what it was like to have my heart pumping in a health inducing way. That in itself was like a gift from heaven. Having said that, on a daily basis pushing myself through my still unnerving dizziness and continual exhaustion did test to the limit my newly discovered resolve. There were also dozens of mornings when the last thing that I wanted to do was exercise and I had to literally drag myself out of bed. But, I knew the alternative.

During my fresher year at university I also came across the work of Anthony Robbins, perhaps one of the most famous people in the area of personal development. At the age of twenty-three Anthony Robbins had been thirty pounds overweight, flat broke, seriously depressed, totally alone and living in a tiny apartment without even a kitchen sink. In one year he had achieved his ideal weight (that part took only thirty days), become a millionaire, found and married the woman of his dreams, and created for himself all the things that he believed he needed to be happy.

Twenty years later, Anthony Robbins was now worth well over 500 million dollars and changing countless lives for the better every day. His tapes and books were sold worldwide, and his seminars infamous for their impact on people, however severe their challenges. His list of famous clients was also pretty impressive, including Presidents of the United States, Princess Diana, Andre Agassi, and numerous other sports people, musicians and other media personalities. Much of what Anthony Robbins taught mirrored my own experiences. He called his main philosophy "Personal Power," which he defined as the ability to take action, something that I felt I had already been doing rather a lot of. The most exciting thing for me about Anthony Robbins was the audio learning programmes that he had produced. Rather than listening to music while I was resting, I could now feed my mind life-changing information. Once again, the power of my focus meant that every minute in my day was being utilised.

Because of the countless hours I spent listening to personal development tapes, over the course of several months I literally re-wrote the part of my brain that processed life. Rather than responding to events in the same negative way I had automatically learnt from my family, I started to choose my responses and actions. People around me soon started to notice the difference, actually asking how it was that I was so happy. Well, it certainly wasn't the events of my life!

Unfortunately, despite my rapidly growing love for the wonders of the human psyche, my university work was rarely what I hoped it would be. Much of what was taught did not even come to close to what I was learning in my spare time. The general conclusion of my professors seemed to be that change is something that is very difficult, and that in many cases the best available option is masking symptoms using dangerous drugs. Yet, such approaches did not seem to be of benefit to anyone I knew who was using them, including my own family members. As far as I was concerned many of my lecturers, although supposedly at the leading edge, were still living in the Ice Age of understanding.

Apart from the frustrations of my course, my only real low time during my fresher year was going home for holidays. The sudden loss of my new life always hit me hard, but I used the time as best I could, continually working on my health and myself. In the Christmas holiday I started to write some articles on personal growth and ME, and I spent the Easter period working towards my summer exams. It was then that I also took another massive step along my healing path.

Iain telephoned one day towards the start of the holidays to ask if I was interested in going on a yoga retreat with him the coming weekend. I had no time to think about it; he needed a decision right away to ensure he secured me the place that had just come up. Despite the retreat entailing eight hours of yoga in two days, massively more than I would normally have dreamt of attempting, I went with my gut reaction: yes. Coming off the phone, a part of me said that I was crazy and that I would never be able to handle it, but I knew by now that I just had to follow life's guidance.

The weekend turned out to be one of my best in years. At times I did get extremely tired and the physical challenge was truly great. But, I took regular rests throughout the day, and although I missed out on much of the social interaction, it felt incredible to sweat out my inner pain as I entered postures I could only have dreamed of performing just a few months previously. Yoga was rapidly becoming my new love.

By the time I returned to university for the summer term, I was feeling truly on top of my recovery and living in anticipation of the great possibilities held by the summer. I knew that moving home for three months would be hard, but I was getting ever closer to reaching my dreams. I hoped that I might be able to start playing golf again, have a holiday, and perhaps even get a job and begin to live a totally normal life. All I had to do first was get through summer exams. Last year's nightmare was still lingering in my mind, but I reasoned that things would surely be different this time. If only.

CHAPTER 16: ALL IN THE MIND? (SUMMER 2000)

Do not weep;
Do not wax indignant.
Understand.
Baruch Spinoza

I worked in the period leading up to exams in the same way I had worked for my A-levels: I sorted my notes, worked through past questions, and then in the final days planned to commit the information to memory. I took confidence in the fact that I only had to average 40% in each paper, and if I didn't, there were always the re-sits. In addition, first year results had no influence on my final degree anyway. There was no logical reason why my body would be over stressed. Having made it through the first paper with ease, I was further reassured.

As I lay in bed the night before my second exam, my head was a cocktail of facts about the next day's paper. With the various flavours swirling around me I simply couldn't switch off; I had forgotten how to sleep. It seems that, in the middle of the night, things that in the light of day can be clearly seen for what they are, irrational thoughts, are somehow able to smother even the most logical parts of the human mind. I just couldn't stop the movies of things falling apart playing in my head. The more I saw them, the more disturbed I felt, and so the more I was sucked in. Nothing I tried seemed to break the loop; even my usual sleep-inducing meditations and taking an early hour walk around the tower block where I lived, failed. I ended up having a dreadful night's sleep and becoming increasingly nervous and agitated with every long hour that passed.

By the morning I was in a really bad way. I felt like hell, and feeling like hell was something I had a lot of terrifying memories of. I had entered what I would soon call the ME state of mind. With that shift in state, months of progress suddenly disintegrated, and thousands of hours of dedicated hard work fell away. I crashed, and it hurt. It really hurt.

However, I didn't have time to cry or feel depressed; I had an exam that afternoon. How the hell was I going to do it? If I missed the paper, then I would have to take re-sits in September, meaning I would be unable to relax all summer. But, far scarier than that, for apparently no reason, my health was rapidly deteriorating again. For the first time in nearly a year I could again see only the dark.

Thankfully, just as it had rescued me before, the drive of my spirit once again kicked back in and I did end up sitting the paper, along with the rest. But, although not nearly as difficult as the previous year, surviving did once again take incredible determination. This time there were also other complications; I just about had the energy to cook, but I needed food from somewhere. With my family two hundred miles away, who was going to do my shopping? Luckily, I did have something this time that I had not before: friends. But, in asking for the help that I knew was there, I had to learn an important lesson: my masculine ego had to come down.

In the middle of this period a surprising thing happened. One of my close friends, Becky, came around for an evening to keep me company. Seeing that I was tense and obviously stressed out, she gave me a massage. The result was that for the first time since Emily, a member of the opposite sex touched me in a sexual way. Despite how ill I was, feeling Becky's hands caress my skin I started to feel more alive than I had in years. My body, which for so long had been something that I had hated inhabiting, almost vibrated with energy, as if it was singing with relief. I was letting someone into my world and it felt incredibly good.

My experiences of this period were a mixture of the agony of trying to study and take exams, making the short walk to the kitchen where I had to face severe dizziness if I was to have anything to eat that day, and Becky. In the middle of these bizarre circumstances, Becky fell for me. We had been close friends all year and, now she had broken up with her long-term boyfriend, there became space in her life. It was growing close to Becky that made those weeks so much more bearable than the year before. There was something about being loved and touched that was very nourishing for my soul.

Once exams were over, all my close friends, except Becky, had returned home. We both decided to stay another three weeks, right up until we had to vacate our accommodation. In time I moved into Becky's flat, and in doing so made probably my greatest distinction about ME. Once I had a change of environment, my health quickly improved back to where it had been before the exams. This reminded me of how I had started to feel better after my A-levels. What was more, going to university and breaking the mental patterns of living at home had also helped increase my energy. But what did all this mean? Was ME all in the mind? That couldn't be the case; my dietary changes, meditation, yoga and qigong had clearly been the source of my limited recovery. However, the effect of changing my mental space could also not be denied.

For the first time I really started to look at my thoughts. The more I analysed them, the more I was stunned by their neurosis. Even after all the work I had done on myself, it seemed that negativity and anxiety about my health constantly plagued my mind. I also started to discover that a lot of what were ME symptoms were identical to symptoms of anxiety. This was a really hard thing for me to accept. Any comment about ME having a psychological element until this point brought out an angry side of my character that was seen very rarely. However, I could no longer deny the effect of my state of mind on my illness.

If my body was in a constant state of panic, and so my adrenals were firing adrenaline the whole time, then I clearly would feel exhausted. Serious tension would also explain my still persistent hypoglycaemia. In addition, if I was spending so much time in my mind disconnected from the world and not in present reality, then no wonder I often felt dizzy and spaced out. Although I didn't for a moment question the realness of my symptoms, they were far too terrifying for me to ever forget, I started to realise that it was the fact that they were terrifying which was part of the problem; the fear itself was adding to my dis-ease.

Reflecting upon my new insights, I knew I still wasn't seeing the whole picture. I therefore applied my transformation formula from the past: I got as much information as I could and immersed myself in it. My uncle was the first person who I went to with my new discovery. I got some very profound advice.

Iain explained, "Everyone has this part of their mind (in Freudian terminology what is called the "super-ego," popular psychology often calls it the "inner-critic/judge"), that is constantly chattering away; most people spend their lives governed by it. However, you are not these thoughts, for if you were you couldn't witness them. Imagine that you are in a room where there is a television playing the news. Now, as you know, the news is rarely an accurate portrayal of reality; it is a list of all the bad events that have happened in the day. This part of your mind is like that. It's constantly telling you about all the terrible things that might happen, most of which are totally fictitious. Although such thoughts may always be there, you do not have to listen to them, for they only have the power that you give. You can watch the news and feel really depressed, or you can just see it for what it is, bad news."

This sounded great, all I had to do was stop listening to the chatterbox in my mind and I would be happy and healthy! As I was later to find out, this chatterbox is one of the main sources of human misery, and it is the same thing that many spiritual searchers are trying to transcend. I decided that I was unlikely to beat it in a few days, but surely a week or two would be enough? More seriously, I realised it would take time; but as I reminded myself, all great journeys start with a single step, and I was about to really begin the search of a lifetime: to find out who I truly am underneath the gabbling of my mind.

Upon reading further, and continuing to meditate on my new ideas, my understanding deepened. What I had started that night nearly two years ago, in committing to finding the answers to ME, was beginning to show me things that I had probably not been ready to see then. For quite some time I had been questioning the sanity of not only myself, but also of everyone around me. I just couldn't understand why so many people lived lives that they hated and why human beings worldwide seemed to be in such a mess. In answering these questions, the powerful writings of the spiritual teacher A. H. Almaas in many ways deepened my concern.

Reading that our personality, what we think is who we are, is an illusion, that it is simply a mere construct of our family conditioning, was a shocking thing to me. What I intuitively feared, that most people are totally out of touch with their essential selves, was written right there in front of me in a way that held more truth than I wanted to admit. The idea that we are not who we think we are also posed rather an interesting question in my mind: then who are we? The answer that I read spoke to me profoundly: at our essence we are all that we seek in the outside world; we are infinite joy, love, truth, compassion, power and understanding.

With such insights, the world that throughout my illness had created such serious depression in me was starting to make more and more sense. However, my neurosis was in many ways just growing. Everywhere I looked I was questioning reality, including my own existence; the more I did so, the crazier I felt I was becoming. Fearing what my new friends might think, I kept my questions about human consciousness to myself. In fact, I rather envied them, in many ways I wished I didn't know what I did; it appeared a hell of a lot easier to just be able to go about everyday life.

In discovering what I had about the personality and its attempts to provide on the outside what we have lost touch with on the inside, I assumed that I would now be free from mine. Alas, it seems that the intellectual understanding is rarely enough, for I was about to make one of the most personality driven decisions of my life.

Becky was continuing to fall for me and, although I was attracted to her sexually, I knew that she was very different from the kind of the woman I truly wanted. She was special in her own way, and quite beautiful, but she just did not have the depth of being I truly desired. However, the more she fell for me and told me how she felt, the more tempted I became. I somehow knew that, even though I was being totally honest with her and telling her that I didn't want a long-term relationship, it was a bad idea. Yet, I was nearly twenty years old and still as much of a virgin as I had been at fifteen. I reasoned: what harm would it do to just have casual sex together? No one would get hurt, I told myself, especially if I was honest.

I agonised over how to handle the situation for several days, and in the end temptation won; I decided to go with my desires. I ignored the inner voice that had guided me so valuably through the past two years. In doing so I ignored my own soul. As I was soon to learn, this is never a wise move. Interestingly, although I thought my hesitation was that I didn't want to use and hurt Becky, she wasn't the only one that got hurt.

Soon I had lost my virginity and I immediately became addicted to the feelings of intimacy that accompany having sex. It just felt incredible to be so close to another human being. For our final few weeks in Wales, before returning home to our respective parents who lived about an hour's drive from each other, Becky and I made love three or four times a day, stayed up late watching films, and slept in until the early afternoon. Due to us being overheard by Becky's flatmates on a number of occasions, I also earned a reputation as a bit of a stud. With my serious lack of experience this was quite a surprise, although I wasn't complaining!

However, despite the fun that I was having, I was glossing over how I truly felt, and I had to live with that. This was especially difficult for me considering how much I prided myself in my integrity. Although Becky knew the circumstances, as far as I was concerned I should have had more control. I knew that it was my growing ambition to impact on the world around me and to help others find out who they truly are and what they are really capable of. Believing that I was taking the easy option was at times creating an inner civil war. "How can I teach this stuff if I don't use it?" I kept telling myself.

Thankfully, the universe was, as always, still guiding me; I was about to get just the experience I needed. The previous summer, Iain

99

and Renate had been on the Anthony Robbins seminar "Unleash the Power Within," and, this year, yours truly was attending. In exchange for one hundred and twenty hours work in his office over the summer, Iain had lent me the money. A great focus of the seminar was on overcoming fear. I reasoned that with my new insights about my health this was exactly what I needed. Of course, being the biggest seminar of its kind in the world, there was going to be an equally big metaphor. So, the first night I would end up really experiencing the neurosis of my mind: I was going to walk across twelve feet of coals burning at two thousand degrees. Yes, I was planning on doing a fire-walk!

CHAPTER 17: FACING THE FEAR

The way this works is, you do thing you are scared shitless of, and
you get the courage after you do it.
Three Kings

Standing in queue with 5,000 other people, waiting to get into Wembley Arena for the start of the seminar, I realised that the Mean Fiddler, where I had played guitar with Sugarkane only two years earlier, was just around the corner. My experiences in the music industry seemed like a lifetime away; they almost felt like memories of a different person. I guess in many ways they were.

As the crowds of people slowly edged forwards, my internal state was a combination of excitement at being in the presence of one of my favourite teachers, and also a growing fear at the thought of the weekend's insane schedule. Anthony Robbins was well known for his desire to teach for excessively long periods of time without stopping, and this meant that over the next three-and-a-half days there was going to be around forty hours of training. This was more hours of energy than I would normally use in a week.

Playing more on my mind than before was also the thought of the fire-walk. I knew from promotional materials that 99.99% of people who had attended the seminar had done it, but of course the chatterbox in my mind was telling me I was different. It reminded me that the fire-walk was not until around midnight, by which time I would be very drained and my blood sugar levels unusually low. What if I collapsed or wiped myself out for the rest of the weekend? Surely I should just leave early and get some much-needed rest for the following day.

When I had to sign a disclaimer on my registration form, saying that there was no medical reason preventing me from doing the fire-walk, I was again instructed by my chatterbox that this was the perfect opportunity to opt out. What did it really matter anyway, it questioned. Yet, in constant battle with such excuses was a part of me that was determined to go beyond my anxieties. A whole four years of my life had been ruined by what was increasingly looking like an illness with a major psychological component. What if this was an opportunity to finally break free from ME? How could I waste such a chance? I knew that I had to face what I feared; if I didn't, I might spend the rest of my life in the prison that had become my world. But, knowing this in my heart was not enough; I still needed to convince my own mind.

By the time Anthony Robbins had appeared on stage to ecstatic applause, my chatterbox was winning. It had convinced me that just by attending the seminar I had done the most important part; if I really learnt the information, surely that was enough? However, deep down I knew this was rubbish, another attempt by my old limiting patterns at sabotaging my life once again. I knew I couldn't continue living with such excuses and the resultant inner conflict. I had to find the strength to pacify my demons from somewhere.

After a couple of hours of Anthony Robbins's unique teaching style I was starting to fight back. Towering at six foot seven, with his size sixteen shoes, huge frame, and inimitable voice and charisma, he had the entire arena captivated. We were moved by stories of people overcoming adversity and defying the odds in life, whilst at the same time taught the principles of creating a successful life. It was impossible not to be affected by what was being said; the spirit of which was that the human family is capable of so much more than it currently manifests. Who could honestly disagree with such truth?

As the build up continued, all possible means were used to put us in the most positive state possible. Therefore, in the middle of Anthony Robbins's carefully crafted words, every so often the arena would pound with music and many of us jumped up and danced on our chairs. Of course my chatterbox had a few things to say about this. "You won't have enough energy to last," it kept telling me, "Why don't you sit the dancing out?" However, I take little credit for winning this battle. Once it looked like there was a chance I might be doing the fire-walk, my chatterbox kicked back in with, "Well, if you're really going to do this, make damn sure you do the build up properly. If you lose your feet it's really gonna hurt!"

Being told that people have been emotionally traumatised through fire walking, received all sorts of terrible burns, and in fact even died, did not help in my battle. Neither did being reminded that the coals would be two thousand degrees and that we were not to run in case we tripped and got cooked. What was a little bit of a comfort was that of the 750,000 people who had done this particular Anthony Robbins seminar, no one had been seriously injured. The few injuries that had taken place had not been due to the actual fire-walk, but from people stepping on coals that had strayed away from the lanes (and so they came in contact with them when they were not in the appropriate frame of mind). But, as my chatterbox was constantly reminding me, there's a first time for everything!

Everything suddenly became very real a couple of hours before we were due to walk. All 5,000 of us journeyed to a car park behind the arena and witnessed the lighting of the gigantic bonfire that was producing our coals. I knew that in a very short period of time I would be attempting to do something that would test someone in full health to the extreme, something that is, supposedly, impossible. The countless hours I had spent listening to tapes and reading books were one thing, but this was different; this was risking my life. However, I did know that if I succeeded I would re-connect with a resource inside of myself that I had not felt in a long time: my true power. I would also gain an opportunity to hear a new record in my mind, a record other than that of ME. I wanted such a transformation more than anything.

During the final build up, we did a repeated exercise where we would look people in the eye and with every ounce of our self-belief shout, "You're walking tonight, and so am I!" I guess this was designed to convince us that we could, and were, going to partake. It worked! As I screamed out at the people around me, I suddenly realised the truth: I couldn't squander this opportunity. If I went home having given in, how would I live with myself? I would be setting a precedent of fear for the rest of my life. And, was I really willing to pass on an opportunity to defy all those who have ever doubted the power of the human spirit?

Once the time to fire-walk had arrived, the atmosphere in the arena was electric. 5,000 people were together about to face their fears; we were literally going to walk on fire. We half-walked and half-danced behind the arena, clapping our hands in unison. I hate to think what the stewards thought; we must have looked like members of some New Age cult!

As we reached the car park of fear, I saw in the distance the lanes of coal for the first time; they held worrying similarity to a barbecue. I just hoped that there was no meat being cooked, for apart from being a vegetarian, I feared that my feet might be on the menu. With the sound of tribal drums leading our transformations there was a powerfully hypnotic flavour in the air. All around there were screams of ecstasy as people completed their walks and simultaneously took a step closer to their dreams. I prayed that if I screamed it would be for the right reasons.

Yet, as the coals got closer, my sense of humour deserted me and all of a sudden I felt very alone. In the midst of being surrounded by such intense positive emotion, my depression was still managing to lurk its ugly head. I started to think about all the suffering in my life, the pain and fear that seemed to be the centre of my existence. Who was I to think that I could change now? Surely I was stupid to think that I could truly face my fears. Why even try? You are just a weak person born to suffer, the stripping down continued.

It was not my fault, I was told: I had had a hard life; fear and depression were just my destiny. My screwed up family and being hated at school; my years trapped inside a body that at times found it an effort to even walk to the toilet; they were just a taste of the life that had been chosen for me. Imagining a future based on this past, my whole existence just seemed like one big horrible mess. There was no way I could take anymore. I started to feel so much pain and so much fear that I knew I could not go home without walking across those coals. To do so would mean my failure to live out my promise of a year ago, my oath to create the life of my dreams. In doing that I might once again contemplate the ultimate escape. I knew that I could no longer continue to be paralysed by fear and stuck in a life of illness. My whole future came down to the next few minutes. One chance. One decision. All I had to do was turn my back and it would be over. I truly felt like I was once again staring death in the face; or was it destiny?

As this mental fire was burning inside me, I was getting dangerously close to something that was even hotter. Looking around, I saw Anthony Robbins in charge of the coals five lanes across. I needed his help. Pushing through the mass of people to join the queue in front of him, my fear rose to panic. Over the past year listening to his tapes and reading his books I had gained incredible respect for his achievements and ability to take people beyond their fears. If anyone could help me break free it was surely he?

Just as the panic in my mind reached fever pitch, my turn arrived. There was mutiny inside; I couldn't do it. My fear was too much. I just couldn't find what I needed within in me. I made the most fatal mistake. I looked at what I feared. I focused on the glowing coals in front of me. My chatterbox had won. It was over.

"I can't do this," I said, turning away.

My heart was in pieces. How was I going to live with myself? Could I really carry the pain and fear inside me for much longer? Thank God the universe was, as always, watching. Before I could destroy myself any further, I heard Tony speak to me.

"You are so ready for this," was all he said.

Suddenly the most extraordinary thing happened. I started to punch the air and scream at the top of my voice; an eruption of power began unleashing from within me. Like an energy that had lain dormant for years, my spirit exploded. The neuroses of my mind simply vanished, and before I knew it I was storming across 2,000 degrees of burning coals barefoot. Seconds later I was on the other side jumping like a mad man, feeling more self-belief than I had known was possible. Joining in the celebrations of my fellow participants, it started to hit me what I had just done: I had faced my fears; I had stood up to the monsters in my mind. What did this mean was now possible for my life? Would I now be free from ME?

For the drive back to my B&B that night, courtesy of my new friend Carl (walking on fire has a unique ability to initiate some rapid male bonding) there was only one thing I could say, "I can't believe I just did that!" I now knew what it must feel like to take drugs. No wonder people become addicts, I thought to myself. I could quite easily have spent the rest of my life feeling that way.

The rest of the weekend was spent learning and experiencing much of the contents of Anthony Robbins's tapes and books. Although I wasn't aware of it at the time, in the midst of this, a seed was being planted in my mind. My heart began to realise that at some point in the future, I, like Anthony Robbins, would lead seminars. I had finally witnessed a medium by which I would be able to dramatically impact upon people's lives and make a difference in the world. It was taking me a while to get used to the idea, but there had been no accidents in my life. I was not born to go to hell and back simply for the journey. All that had happened to me had been part of my education. Eventually I would graduate from the school of life, and it would then be time to teach. However much time I might spend trying to deny it and struggling to fit in and be normal, normality was not my destiny. There would only be so long I could continue to deny the person I really am.

Unfortunately, upon returning home, ME was still very much a part of my existence. But, despite the seminar having not directly impacted upon my health, it had still been of massive benefit to me. For one thing it had radically increased my sense of self-belief and expectations from life. These were changes that would only continue to grow over the coming years.

Moving home for the summer months was immensely difficult, even with all my new knowledge about influencing human behaviour.

Apart from having no close friends near where I lived, my relations with my family were as challenging as ever. My continuing personal transformation was extremely difficult for certain people to take, and despite my mother's pleas, on a number of occasions I was told I was unwelcome at home. Once again someone that deep down I loved was rejecting me; my silent response was hiding much still unhealed inner pain. Yet, I had no choice but to stick it out. There was to be no escape for now.

Perhaps worse than my family situation, regardless of the massive changes that I had created in my life over the previous two years, I still found my mind flying back to that space where there was only one record playing: the record of illness. It was incredibly painful to see everything I had worked so hard for falling apart once again. I was, however, making progress on several major fronts. Firstly, I was working at Iain's office to pay him back for the seminar and, although I was only doing half days, this was still an undeniable improvement upon the year before in my energy. Secondly, I was using my spare time to start work on these very pages you hold in your hand. Doing so made life just bearable; it was incredibly soothing to put into words the so many emotions still locked in my body.

As I continued battling to break free, on the second attempt I managed to get my driving licence. Within a month of that I had my own car (courtesy of family savings that I had just come into). By the last month of the holidays I had even been to a recording studio to produce some of my own music and played a few holes of golf. Yet, despite once again being able to work and participate in my old hobbies, there was continually a black cloud hanging over me, and it was more than just the fact that I was still chronically ill.

I was a different person now. I was trying to fit back into a life I had departed four years ago and it just wasn't working. If I wanted to feel passionate about my life I was going to have to stop listening to those around me and start paying attention to my own heart. However, my fear of doing so was even greater than my fear of those burning coals had been.

In some ways having an idea of what is really inside of us all and not being able to contact it was worse than not knowing. Knowing the natural happiness in newly born babies only added to this frustration. I knew that we all once felt such joy; that is before we were conditioned to believe that you must do certain things and act certain ways to be loved. Looking at people in our culture who were supposed to be

106

successful, I was only too aware of the illusion of the personality's false wisdom. Most who had reached the top of the mountain of success were either depressed, addicted to some quick fix drug for their pain, or they had jumped off (i.e. they had killed themselves). The only truly happy people I had met, or read about, had found their happiness from turning within and looking to themselves for their own dreams, truth and self-love. Yet, in my journey to do so I was still struggling greatly.

In the middle of this frustrating time, things with Becky and me became even more complicated. She eventually got fed up with my lack of commitment and went back to her former boyfriend. Upon missing her affections, I managed to deceive myself into thinking that I did feel something more for her, even though the truth was that I just missed the intimacy we had shared. With Becky I felt loved, I felt wanted and I felt special. These were needs that hadn't been met for many years. In lying to myself, I declared my commitment to her, and what followed was a time of my life that I could feel very embarrassed about. I continued to have sex with Becky while she was with her boyfriend, convincing myself that in time she would see that I was the one she really wanted. It is amazing how our need to be loved can deceive us, and the more I became frustrated with living at home and being separated from my university friends, the more I acted out of character.

Fortunately, once one of our mutual friends, Nadia, found out what was going on she gave me a proverbial kick in the backside. I am glad to say that I had the courage to listen and immediately ended the affair. Even though Becky did finally decide she wanted to be with me, I had thankfully learnt my lesson and we remained just friends. I had discovered the hard way never again to use relationships to fill my inner emptiness, realising that what can appear like a quick fix never is; it only prolongs feeling the truth. It also prepared me for the kind of relationship that I really deserved. Although I thought at the time that this was many years away, for once my intuition was wrong.

And it was around this point that this book originally finished. Yet, as events unfolded further, it became clear that my health still had much to teach me. For the next few months I worked incredibly hard on producing a first draft of this book, set my mind to what I wanted, and assumed I would never look back. Such is the beauty of a naïve young mind! I still had a lot of growing up to do before I would finally reap the benefits of walking the path less travelled. But, it is interesting to note the influence and power of divine intervention, for although this book was several years from its final completion, even in its creation it had a unique role to play in my life, along with the life of a rather amazing woman. The paths of two searching souls were about to join in a remarkable way.

CHAPTER 18: A DIVINE MEETING (WINTER 2000)

Healing is the way in which separation is overcome.
A Course in Miracles

It was late November and I was settling into my second year in Swansea. Although life was undoubtedly easier again being away from the turmoil of living with my family, the carefree days of my fresher year seemed to be behind me. I was once again struggling with my depression and trying to understand the subtler aspects of existence. In an attempt to fill my inner void, I was attending four or five yoga classes a week and devouring every book on personal transformation I could find; it was making a difference, but it wasn't enough. I knew deep down that I would only truly be happy once I created a way to live as my true self in the world; until then the struggle would continue.

Events with my new housemates were certainly not helping. I had chosen to live with three Christians, for in the absence of discovering anyone my age with genuinely similar interests, I figured that we at least might have some interesting discussions. I guess interesting is one way to describe the interactions that unfolded. Within a few weeks of moving in, the four of us went about redecorating our kitchen. As we carried out our allotted tasks, the apparently controversial topic of religion arose. Before I knew it I was being verbally attacked for many of my deepest held understandings, and in no uncertain terms told that if I didn't turn my life over to God (according to their definition) I would go to hell and experience eternal suffering and damnation. Jesus had died for me, and for this I owed him everything, I was informed. How I could be so blind as not to see this, they questioned.

Although not unfamiliar with such fundamentalism, it did rather shock me coming from three people who I had hoped were to become close friends. I decided not to point out that if/when Jesus returns (there are already a number of people in mental asylums claiming they are he) the chances are that he will be treated with the same hatred as before, most probably this time by the Christians. After all, how will he be distinguished from those alive today that have the same healing powers; those same people labelled as heretics? The whole thing still confused me severely!

The result of our dead-end debate was an uneasy truce. Perhaps the most frustrating thing about my supposed friends was their incredible hypocrisy; on a daily basis our living room was abound with sexist comments and bigotry. I questioned whether this was really the behaviour of higher spiritual beings.

And in this vein life went on, with university work being disposed of as fast as possible (a little bit too fast as I was to discover a few months prior to summer exams) so that I could continue to work on myself in every way possible. There were now few books left in either the local or university libraries that fell into my realm of interest that I had not read, yet I kept on studying, expanding my vision as rapidly as I could.

A month prior to Christmas I had an article published in a psychology journal, expressing my view that although I knew ME to be a very real physical illness, and not "all in the mind," my experience was showing the key to recovery as being psychological attitude. I passionately expressed my discoveries about the potential for human beings to transform their lives, including the apparently incurable ME. The response was encouraging, with a number of sufferers contacting me expressing how the article had touched them; several people even requested to read a working version of this book (which I sent to them). Again, the response to this was powerful and, before I knew it, people were looking to me for advice on how to recover. It felt incredible to use my experiences to help.

Interestingly, the ME charities were less excited by my ideas, basically telling me that there was no known way to heal the body of ME and that the only course of action was just to wait. They also suggested that, so as to avoid what they saw as my inevitable relapse, I read several books on the findings of research into ME. I already had, including the books written by the person concerned. Let's just say that they had their uses, although firewood would be cheaper! Such lack of support for my ideas essentially made me even more determined, proving even further I had a message that needed to be heard.

In the midst of the ongoing frustrations that had become my life, there was one particular person who responded to my article, and subsequently my book, who stuck in my mind. Her name was Catherine, and the following e-mail touched me deeply:

Hi again,

Almost 7pm - just about to go home, but couldn't go without letting you know I have been able to open the file myself (am very pleased with myself!) and skimmed through yr bk several hours ago. I started to read the end bit first - habit of mine - in the college comp room and it moved me to tears, which I just let flow I was so absorbed.

Something personal I want to share with you, as you have been so brave yourself in bearing your soul in yr bk. Hope you don't mind. I have been feeling really low lately as it's that time of year - everyone in couples and those who aren't are out partying successfully (usually at Christmas) getting together with someone new. As you know, and explained so well, I feel upset that I can't do that, and have been really wanting to be part of a relationship (I'm a Libran!). I have also been really depressed that all my friends are getting engaged etc all around me, and at 31, I had been thinking that it was my illness that was preventing me from having one. Today I found the answer in your bk. I am still looking outside of myself to "cure" what is inside - lack of self-love. It's a biggy for me, which I thought I had solved - thanks to Louise Hay and her many books (yes, they were the first things I turned to, actually 5yrs before I got ME). Anyway, I wanted to say thank you for my light bulb moment. Just knowing that the answer lies within me and not me finding someone has relieved so much sadness and anxiety, it's amazing.

I also wanted to offer you my services, so to speak, as I feel a connection due to our experience (so similar despite the fact you are bags younger than me). Something I discovered this year is Reiki. Don't know if you know anything about it? Basically, it's hands on healing. I am qualified Reiki II, so when you are in Surrey and have an hour to spare, if I can get to you, I will give you a free Reiki session. I am taking your book with me to Holland on my hols (28/12 to 3/1) - wanted to be out of the country to see in New Year - although I'd much rather abandon my multi-store memory model psychology essay and read it now, but I'd regret it come the deadline in Jan.

Could go on all night - but won't. Take good care of yourself. Thinking positive thoughts for you.

Best wishes.

Catherine

*PS home tel is 0208*** **** should you need Reiki or a stranger to talk to over Christmas! (gave up mobile when ditched job)*

PPS I don't usually give out my tel no so easily, but after what I've read so far, I really feel I can trust you.

Despite her clear challenges, Catherine came across as so courageous and open to the guidance of the universe in her e-mails. She was just the kind of person I wanted as a friend, and I sincerely hoped she might become so. Her reading my article had been what some would call a coincidence, and what I would call divine intervention. Only the week before Catherine read it she had told Joy, a fellow student of hers, that she was working on recovering from ME. Joy had stumbled across my article when flicking through the magazine and given it to Catherine. Had Catherine not told Joy she was ill, had my article been published in the earlier addition (as it was originally meant to be), had Joy not read the magazine, or not mentioned it to Catherine, well my life might have been very different. Another piece of divine intervention meant that Iain had offered me his and Renate's London apartment for the first week in January while they were away. As Catherine happened to also be free we arranged to meet for dinner on the Friday night.

The night before our meeting I called Catherine to make arrangements. The moment I heard her voice I felt an instant connection. I couldn't work out what it was, but I felt like I had known her years. Through reading my book, Catherine knew my deepest fears and my darkest moments, yet she still wanted more. To have another human being know so much about my life and still want to connect with me felt fantastic. Catherine and I laughed and chatted together for well over an hour, the conversation only ending due to my needing to get to bed early so as to rest before my morning's work at Iain's office the following day.

Time is a relative thing, and the next morning just seemed to last forever. Thinking that at least an hour or so had passed, I would look at my watch to notice that it had only been another ten minutes. By the time 2:00 arrived my patience was running out, and I breathed a sigh of relief as I rushed back to Iain and Renate's apartment to get a couple of hours sleep before preparing the vegetables for the dinner I was cooking. I tried to ignore the fact that Catherine had eaten in many of the best restaurants in the world due to her past career as a travel marketer, and just focused on doing what I could with my humble chicken stir-fry.

As I walked to meet Catherine at Warwick Avenue tube station, I had no idea what she would look like. Would she be tall or short, fat or thin? Would I even recognise her? I only knew that she would be wearing a black coat and trousers, a lilac jumper and a red hat. Looking around the tube station, waiting to have my questions answered, I heard her gentle voice behind me.

"Alex?" I was greeted by a slim, extremely beautiful woman, with the most incredible smile, tightly wrapped in a thick winter coat against the chilling January air. Catherine looked divine.

A divine meeting

Before I knew it we had walked back to Iain's apartment, cooked dinner, and started eating. I just couldn't believe how much we had in common. Apart from sharing my passion for music, Catherine loved the same books, practised yoga, meditated, had a passion for personal and spiritual development, and she was even on the same nutritious eating plan.

However, despite feeling engrossed in the conversation and so powerfully attracted to this incredible being, I made sure that I kept careful watch of my feelings. I knew that there was no way a woman of this beauty and magnitude would be romantically interested in someone my age; I would have to wait at least five or six years before I would even stand a chance with a woman in her early thirties. In fact, the more Catherine told me about her life, it amazed me that someone like her would even be spending the evening with someone like me.

Catherine had grown up in Twickenham, and after finishing school had put herself through college. Upon graduating, she had moved to the Canary Islands, where she had lived for several years with her then boyfriend, before eventually returning to England when their relationship ended. For several years after she had travelled to various exotic locations around the world as part of her job. Fourteen months ago Catherine had developed ME and had been forced to give up her job as a consequence. Having worked with persistence and determination to create her own recovery, using many of the same methods that I had, Catherine had recently made enough improvement in her health to return to full time education, and was now at the University of Surrey, studying psychology and counselling.

Yet, it wasn't Catherine's colourful past, or her inner or outer beauty that attracted me to her; it wasn't even all the things that we had in common, or the fact I felt like I had known her forever. It was something far subtler and far more delicate; it was something so precious, but also so simple. It was her incredible trust in the process of life; it mirrored so perfectly my most highly prized value.

Dinner flew by, and soon Catherine and I were sitting on the sofa together discussing my book. I was so entranced by Catherine's aura that I struggled to hear much of what I am sure was highly valuable feedback that she gave me. However, there was one comment that instantaneously penetrated my trance.

In her beautiful voice Catherine half whispered, "You know it's probably a good thing that you live in Wales."

My mind raced. Why was that? Did this mean she felt something

113

more for me, that perhaps I wasn't the only one concealing their emotions? Surely not, I reasoned with myself. I had to be misinterpreting. Still, I needed to make sure. As I responded, I desperately attempted to conceal just how intensely I wanted to know what she was thinking.

"Why is that?" I tried to casually comment.

"Oh, nothing," Catherine blushed, quickly changing the subject.

What was going on? My mind was in massive conflict, torn between logic and emotions. As far as I was concerned, all sense of logic suggested that there was no way Catherine was interested in anything more than friendship. I was eleven years younger, I had barely stepped outside my home country; and I was still relatively ill, very skinny and had a virtually shaven head! Catherine, on the other hand, was a mature woman used to men with careers and money; this was not to mention the fact that she was absolutely stunning. Yet, despite all this logic, my emotions somehow told me there was something deeper between us. Still, I was not ready to gamble my heart on such a whim.

After a few more inner battles trying to understand the complexities of Catherine's beautiful mind, I settled on the conclusion that she really had meant nothing by her passing comment. It seemed too dangerous to even contemplate falling in love with someone as incredible as Catherine. It would surely be futile and ruin the chances of a good friendship, I told myself. After years of practice I did what I was good at, I ignored my feelings.

Before I knew it three hours had shot by, and it was nearly time for Catherine to go. I desperately hoped to see her again and was searching for a way to arrange another meeting, although this was going to be difficult; I was supposed to be driving back to Wales in a few days. While I continued to hunt for the right words, Catherine made my already confused heart skip a few more beats.

"It's nearly 10:00, and I don't want to travel on the tube too late on my own. But, I feel we still have so much to talk about. I also promised to give you a Reiki session in return for all that you have done for me through your book. How would you feel about me staying the night?"

I couldn't believe my ears! Did this mean I was going to be able to spend more time with this incredible woman? However, the sleeping arrangements crossed my excited mind; I desperately needed to get a good night's sleep after a long week struggling with my energy at Iain's office.

114

"You realise there is only one bed, and at my height I can't really sleep on the sofa," I cautiously replied, desperately hoping Catherine didn't think I was trying anything on. "That's fine," Catherine replied, "I trust you."

"Holy shit," I thought to myself. I'm about to share a bed with the woman of my dreams! "Just don't get an erection," I told myself, "Otherwise this could be very embarrassing!"

A few minutes later Catherine was laying her hands on my energy centres giving me Reiki. Receiving Reiki from Catherine was so very different to healing sessions I had experienced in the past; I felt like she was giving so much more than just healing energy. However much I tried to deny it to myself, there was an incredibly deep connection developing between the two of us.

As Catherine finished giving me Reiki twenty-minutes later we shared our experiences. Catherine explained that she had also felt an incredible bond, and asked if she could give me a hug. My mind started to race again. What was happening to me? I was not used to this sort of thing in my life. Just the night before I had experienced the most incredible loneliness trying to get to sleep. After the failure of my usual yogic relaxation exercises, I had only eventually managed to enter the world of dreaming by imagining myself being held in the arms of my spiritual guides. Here I was now, only a day later, with the woman of my dreams. It was like my prayers had been answered.

As Catherine and I held each other I felt slightly uncomfortable with being so close to someone to whom I was so attracted, and yet convinced I would never be able to be in a relationship with. It was also getting harder to ignore my feelings; more and more of me just wanted to throw caution to the wind and tell Catherine how I felt, to share with her the love that I could feel growing inside me. Yet, years of rejection had taken their toll, and I wasn't sure I could handle being hurt again.

After taking it in turns to get ready for bed, we climbed into our separate sides and I put the light out. Lying there, supposedly going to sleep, my mind was doing somersaults, my body felt like it was plugged into the mains, and my heart was pumping a million times a minute. Of the thousands of ideas whirling around my mind, one did offer me some comfort; perhaps one day a woman like this could possibly fall in love with me. Such love would surely change me forever.

As I continued to focus on a distant future experiencing the love of a woman like Catherine, she once again added to my disbelief, nervously asking, "Would you like to hug again?"

"Erm.... OK," I replied, not quite sure what else to say.

We tentatively moved towards each other, both aware that it was dark and we were wearing rather less than we would have ideally chosen. Due to the unexpected nature of our circumstances neither of us had pyjamas, and so my T-shirts and our respective underwear were all that was on offer.

"Your heart is racing. Are you OK?" Catherine questioned as we gently held each other.

"Oh, I'm fine," I replied, slightly embarrassed. "It always does that," I continued, hoping to divert attention from the passion that was building inside of me.

While Catherine and I continued to hold each other, my emotions entered further uncharted territories. The way I was feeling was so unlike the teenage crushes and burning desires to have sex I had known in the past; all I wanted to do with Catherine was savour every moment and make it last forever. Everything about her was perfect; stroking her face and caressing her soft skin I felt pure bliss. I desperately wanted to kiss Catherine and feel her lips embracing mine. However, up until now we could just have been two people holding each other; any more would be crossing a line that she might not want to cross with me. I was in a serious dilemma. Should I wear my heart on my sleeve, yet risk losing all that we had; or should I play it safe? It felt a million miles away from fire-walking, yet so many of the emotions were the same. I knew what I wanted and there was only one thing stopping me: fear.

Before I had time to reason my way around the situation, my heart took over and spoke for me. Without even deciding to do so, I found myself leaning forward and gently kissing Catherine's lips. As Catherine passionately kissed me back, I connected to heaven for the first time in my life. I had been touched by an angel.

I don't know how long we lay there in each other's arms kissing, it felt like only a moment, but it was probably nearer to several hours. Holding Catherine close to me, feeling her heart beating next to mine and hearing her soft voice whispering in my ear, it sent me to places I had never been. To gaze into her deep blue eyes was like seeing right to the centre of her soul. I was in heaven, and I didn't want to come back to earth, ever!

However, come back to earth I had to. Eventually we decided

(actually Catherine decided and I pretended I was thinking the same thing) that we had better get some sleep or we would both feel awful the next day. Try as we might though, I don't think either of us slept a wink that night. As far as I was concerned, I had waited my whole life to meet this woman and I wasn't willing to waste my time with needless tasks such as sleeping!

The next morning we eventually got up and had breakfast. Each time I saw Catherine I had to double blink. I still couldn't believe this amazing woman was falling in love with me! She was no longer just an angel; she was my angel. I somehow knew that together we would learn to fly.

As I waited that morning for Catherine to return from a trip home for more clothes, I cleared my schedule for the next couple of days and also called a couple of my closer friends to share my incredible news. It was interesting to note that there were those that were extremely sceptical. After all, I was reminded, "Eleven years is a huge age difference, especially when you are young." I just took such ideas as a sign of people not truly knowing me. My mum was also a bit shocked, but ultimately supportive; I have a feeling that she had given up any aspirations of me living a "normal" life several years previously!

In the evening Catherine and I went to the cinema to see the Bruce Willis film "Unbreakable." Its key message of listening to life's guidance was rather poignant. I held Catherine's hand on the way to the cinema, put my arm around her during the film, held her hand on the way back, and we once again lay in each other's arms all night. I just didn't want to let her go; I had waited so long to be in love like this and it felt unbelievably good.

But, in a few days things were going to have to change, for I would need to return to university. Thankfully, although being head over heels in love, I still had a firm grip on reality. My feelings for Catherine were growing by the day, yet I also knew that I had to continue with my journey, which for now was over two hundred miles away. I put my trust in the powers that be, and knew that if we were meant to last the distance, then last the distance we would.

So as to save living costs, Catherine had moved home while she was at university, and just before returning to Wales I had the pleasure of meeting her family. For many months to come their house became my home away from Wales. For their kindness at a time when I felt in many ways homeless, I was immensely grateful. It was an amazing feeling to know that I had a soft place to fall, something that had been lacking for most of my life.

In the months leading up to Easter, Catherine and I visited each other as much as we could and, when apart, we both continued doing all that we could to heal ourselves. Yet, despite my continued efforts and newfound love, my health was in many ways once again worsening. My journey with ME that had already taught me so much still had much to share; I still had some of my worst demons to face.

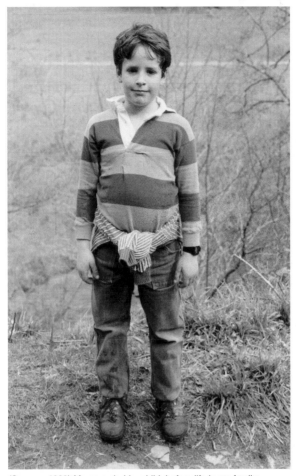

(Summer 1989) Me as a chubby child, before life in my family became more dramatic than a television soap opera.

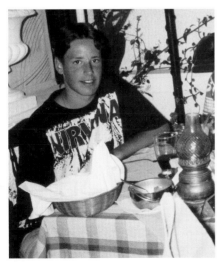

(Summer 1995) On holiday a year before my world fell apart.

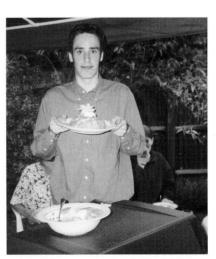

(Summer 1998) At my eighteeth birthday party, trying to ignore the hell that had become my life (holding my sugar/yeast/preservative free birthday cake).

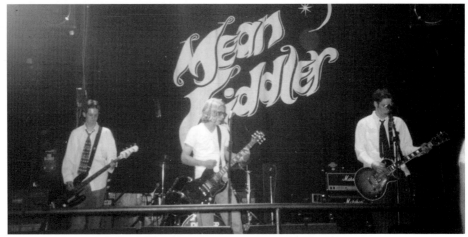

(Summer 1998) On stage with Sugarkane at the Mean Fiddler.

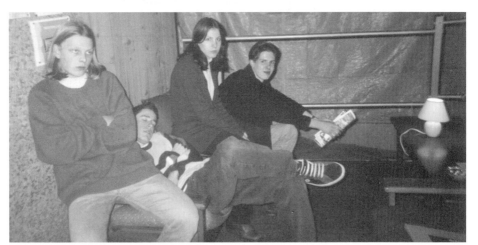

(Summer 1997) Losing my battle against my fragile body in the studio during the mixing of "Opinions EP".

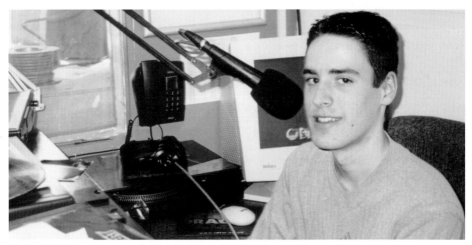

(Spring 2000) Presenting my radio show on "Xtreme Radio" during my first year at University.

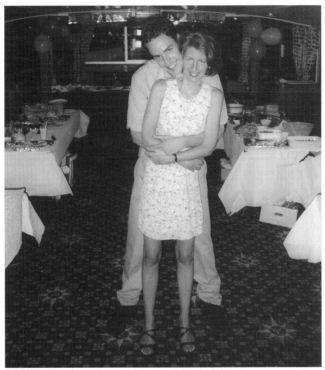

(Summer 2001) Catherine and I at a friend's birthday party.

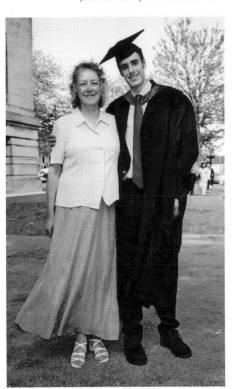

(Summer 2002) Mum and I at my graduation.

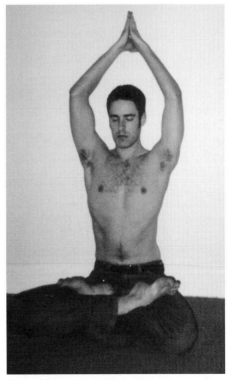

(Spring 2003) An image I yearned for after so many long years – peacefully inhabiting a fit and healthy body.

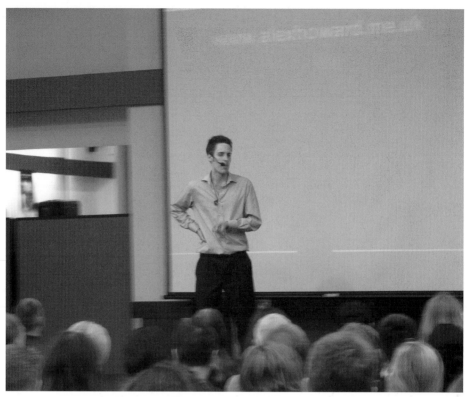

(Spring 2004) On the road promoting this book.

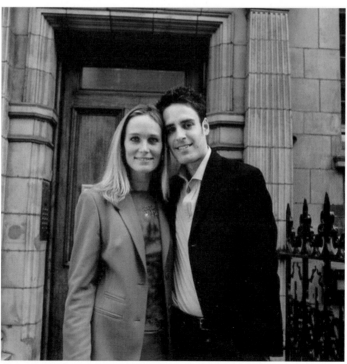

(September 2004) Niki and I proudly at the door to Harley Street.

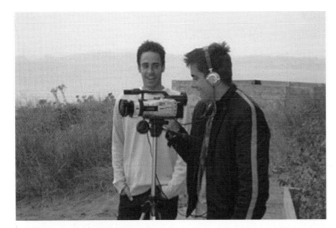

(Summer 2006) Paul and I filming the "Freedom From M.E." DVD.

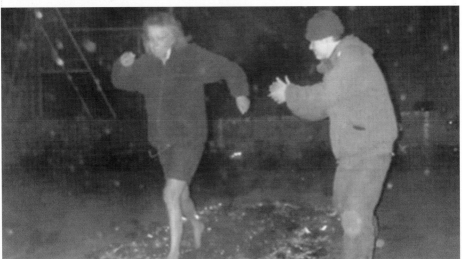

(January 2009) My mother bravely firewalking for The Optimum Health Clinic Foundation.

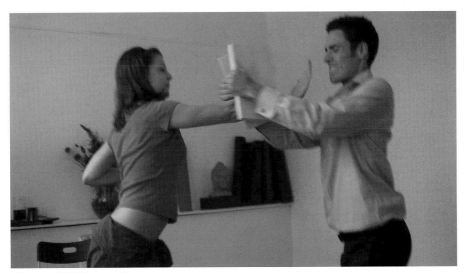

(Summer 2006) Board breaking.

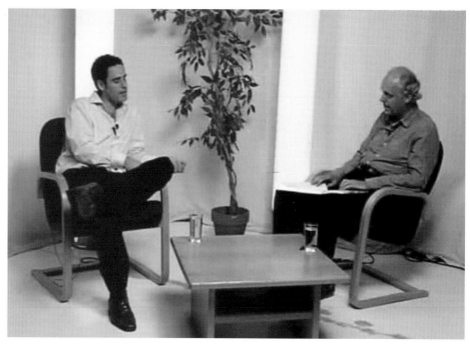

(Autumn 2008) My Uncle Iain and I filming the interview "Healing M.E./C.F.S./Fibromyalgia in the 21st Century."

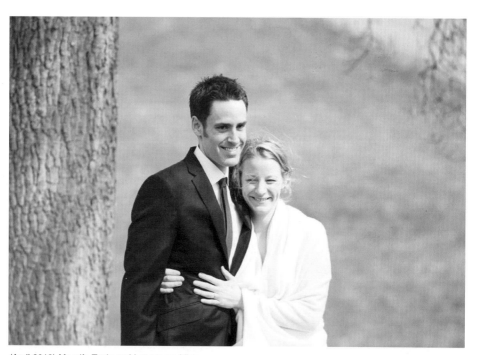

(April 2012) My wife Tania and I at our wedding.

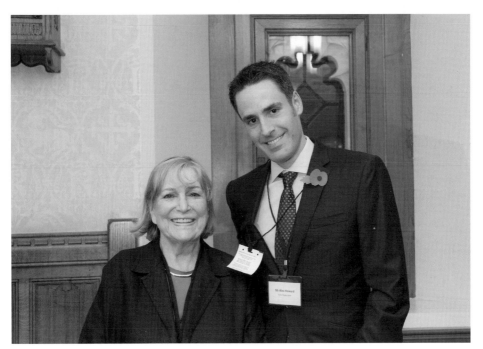

(November 2013) OHC Foundation Patron Shirley Conran OBE and I at the House of Lords.

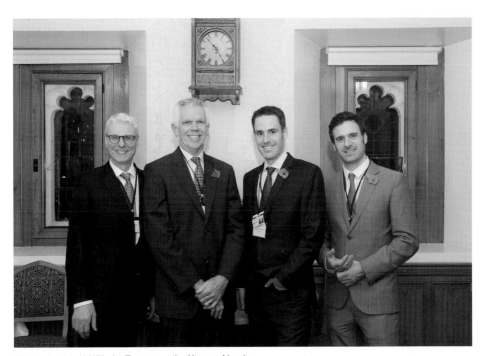

(November 2013) With the Trustees at the House of Lords.

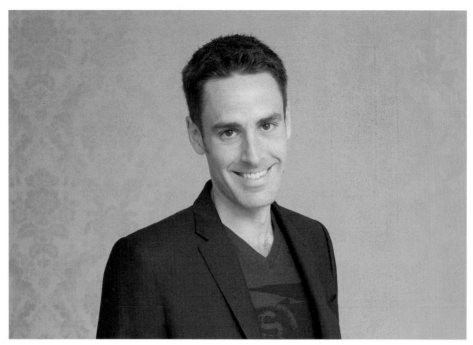

(September 2013) Posing for promo photos.

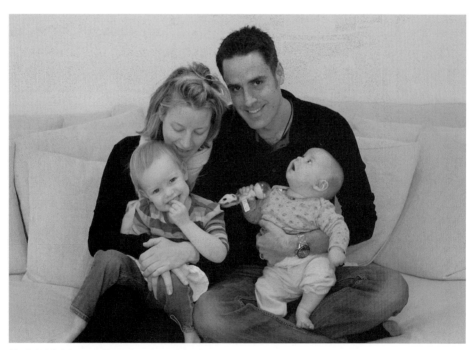

(April 2014) At home with my three beautiful girls.

CHAPTER 19: SHOW ME! (SPRING 2001)

I dance to the tune that is played.
Spanish Proverb

With Christmas behind me, it started to become abundantly clear that areas of my life that had once been rampant with development were now stagnant. Although I was able to force my body to do much of what I wanted it to, I still had severe daily stomach pains and digestive problems, which in many ways seemed to have worsened over previous months. I also still had to sleep every afternoon to get through the day. Years of inactivity and frustration, along with a burning desire to create the life of my dreams, meant I had a pretty high pain threshold, but it eventually became clear to me that motivation was not enough. What I needed was to adopt a new strategy. I therefore got back to the drawing board, and back to some of my contacts in the field of complementary health.

I started off by visiting Dr. Mansfield regarding my digestive problems. As far as he was concerned I was experiencing a regrowth of candida, due to the massive amounts of fruit I had been consuming over the past year in my trial of the healing methods of Natural Hygiene. I consequently went back on his same anti-candida programme I had been on four years previously. The result was pretty ugly as, unlike before, I experienced major die-off symptoms, including far worse than usual dizziness, severe bloating and wind, and fluctuating constipation and diarrhoea. In fact my digestive system was so "confused" that I would often go three or four days without a bowel movement, until my body could take no more and I would then experience extremely painful diarrhoea. Feeling like I had no choice, I just pushed on with life and got done as much as I could. Half-hour-hugs from Catherine when she came to stay did soften the blow and were a beautiful blessing I had not known in the past.

By Easter, I decided that if I kept on feeling this ill, with no tangible improvements, I was going to fail the year at university. The last thing I wanted to do was repeat; the material had been boring enough the first time around. Therefore, once again, I changed my approach, this time going to see Ravi. As far as he was concerned, I didn't have a candida overgrowth and I should stop the anti-fungals immediately. Differing opinions were something I was used to, and in the end the decision was my own. With little to lose, I followed Ravi's advice, for although I believed I did have a candida overgrowth, I knew that passing my exams had to be my priority.

As soon as I stopped the anti-fungals, my die-off symptoms did abate. Yet, there were still no answers as to my continuing health problems. With none of the experts appearing to know what was wrong, I got back to doing my own research and, by experimenting with various balances of protein and carbohydrate, I did make a small amount of progress as far as energy constancy was concerned. Effectively though, my health was going to have to wait for the time being. I had more pressing problems.

With my focus having been so much on my health and healing over the past year, my studies had suffered even more massively than I had realised. With less than ten weeks to go before my second year finals I had almost no notes for the entire year, having only just been able to complete essential assignments. Looking at past papers, I felt like I was reading a foreign language. Regardless of my struggling with my health, it didn't help that the lectures that I had attended were about as exciting as watching paint dry. To say that some of my lecturers lacked a flair for public speaking is a serious understatement; I think many of them lacked a flair for speaking, period.

My university work was not my only cause for concern; my finances were perhaps even less healthy than I was. It reached a head one cold Saturday morning in London when Catherine and I were at the supermarket doing our weekend shopping. I was so broke that I couldn't afford to pay my half; this was after having already reached the overdraft limit on my bank account. The main cause of my situation was the excessive cost of supplements and medical consultations over previous months. But, my purchasing of entertainment in the form of CD's and DVD's, although no different from many of my peers, was also lacking the maturity I showed in other areas of my life.

My response to my academic and financial dilemmas was an interesting one. For the ten weeks prior to summer exams I moved home to eliminate living costs, sold my guitars and all my musical equipment, hardly used my car to save petrol, and got up at 6:30 in the morning to meditate, before spending the day studying. In the evenings, when I was not staying with Catherine, I researched further my health, and also read some books on financial management. In this short period I taught myself the entire second year syllabus for my degree, cleared my overdraft, and actually saved enough money to go on my first holiday in six years. It was on occasions like this that I realised what an incredible gift my illness had been; the self-discipline

I had developed was unbeatable. Little did I know it at the time, but my growing mental muscles would be invaluable in years to come, thankfully for a different reason.

Just prior to exams I attended a life-changing seminar. Its focus was on healing emotional problems caused by one's family, and it aroused within me something I thought had been lost forever. The Sunday evening prior, Iain had called me offering the opportunity to attend for free, the reason being that equal numbers of men and women were needed and there was a shortage of men. "Show me," had become my new motto for life, and therefore, although believing that the only true solution to my family crisis would be that they started considering themselves rather than looking to each other to change, I went along with the guidance of the universe.

The seminar was based on a system of family therapy developed by Bert Hellinger, called "The Orders of Love." Having watched videos of the process prior to attending I thought I had a fairly good understanding of it. I knew that participants would choose members of the audience to represent members of their family, and then place each person spatially in relationship to each other, creating a constellation in the room. The seminar facilitator would subsequently check in with each person to find out what they were experiencing, and from this point feelings would begin to be expressed and changes start to occur. It appeared in the videos to be a powerful experience for everyone involved – those representing family members, those watching from the side, and especially the person whose family was being worked with. Towards the end, the individual would take their place in the system and experience how it was to have their family "healed." The general result for everyone involved seemed to be a lot of trapped emotions being released. That was my intellectual understanding. My actual experience was rather different.

Having watched from the sidelines the first day, at the beginning of the second day I requested to work with my own family system. Doing so was very scary for me, as I knew that I had held onto a lot of negative emotion, throughout both my childhood and my recent years of severe chronic illness. In fact, I could only remember crying on one occasion since I was about twelve (chapter 7), and considering what I had lived through in this time, I had a feeling this was rather a deficit!

Letting my pain go was scary mainly because I had locked it up for a reason: it hurt like hell and I didn't know what to do with it. In fact on many occasions I had felt like I was going to explode, there was so much brimming under the surface. Was I really strong enough to now handle my emotions and release them back to the universe? I did have a pretty strong incentive: I knew that holding emotions in my tissues and organs could very well have been a primary cause of my current health situation. This was another one of those occasions where my commitment to create the life of my dreams had me taking action where with a lesser goal I may have given into my excuses.

With my usual direct and focused frame of mind, I told my story and began to choose participants to represent my family members. After a couple of minutes, Judith, the group facilitator, suggested that I might want to slow down and connect with myself. This idea was about as appealing as jumping off a cliff, for I knew it would mean leaving my usual intellectual experience of the world and entering the rather more unknown realm of feelings. Still, I reasoned that if I was going to do the work, then I needed to do it properly.

Once I had laid out my family, I took my place at the side and watched things unfold. I was pretty struck by the accuracy of what was unfolding. My sister was falling to the ground, my mother struggling to be heard in the middle of my grandmother's taking control, and my stepfather completely lost at what to do. Once again, the magic of the collective consciousness shared by human beings struck me; there was no way these strangers could have guessed with such accuracy how the people I loved felt.

The more the scene in front of me developed, the more I felt my suppressed emotions beginning to rise. I had placed my father at the edge of the constellation for, as he had never been in my life, he didn't seem a relevant part to me. But, within a few minutes he had been moved into the middle and was at the centre of much of what was happening. With this development, I knew my emotions would not be locked away for much longer.

Before I knew it, the time came for me to take my place in my family. As I tentatively got up and moved forwards, tears started to roll down my cheeks. I knew what was coming, and yet for the first time I could remember, I didn't care. By the time I had reached my position I was crying hysterically, my heart was spilling on the floor and my body literally vibrating with the intensity of the emotion that was leaving me. Finally connecting with years of inner pain actually felt unbelievably good; something that had been asleep inside of me was rapidly coming alive: years of unconscious yearning for a supportive family, yearning to have what should have been my birthright, was at last being experienced. I felt like I was having an orgasm of emotion.

As my tears continued to explode, for the first time the true magnitude of living at the centre of my crumbling family touched me. All around me they had been physically and emotionally abusing each other, pushing those they loved to the brink of suicide, all because they hadn't known what else to do. Everyone had been so immersed in their own problems, their own pain and their own personal hell, that they just hadn't known how to help those they deep down loved. I had so desperately wanted to save them, protect them and hold them together. Yet, I hadn't known what to do either. It soothed me deeply to realise, at the deepest level, just how much love was actually underneath the anger and hate that had surrounded my childhood. I dreamed that one day the rest of my family could also feel the truth that I now knew was hidden, especially my sister, George, whom I had barely known since I was eleven.

While my heart continued to release my trapped inner pains, I picked up George from the floor and held her in my arms. I looked at my father next to me, and as I moved tentatively towards him, what was left in my heart erupted and I started to scream with emotion. There were no words, for how do you express deep love, hurt, longing and pain all at once? To have another man next to me, my father, felt incredibly alien. It was almost like suddenly discovering I had a second half to my being. I prayed that one-day I might get used to having such a force in my life.

In time my hysterical crying finally began to slow back down to gentle sobbing, and as it did, the true reality of my childhood sunk in; I had never known my father, and yet I hadn't given it a second thought. I couldn't even begin to comprehend what I had missed out on, how much I had to catch up. My whole life half of my heritage had been stolen from me. For the first time ever it really hit me: I have a father.

Eventually my gentle sobbing also ceased, and left inside of me was for the first time a genuine desire to know my real father, to connect with someone who I should never have been separated from. However, my heart told me that now was not the time for such reunion. But, one day, I prayed, this would change; one day I might meet my dad.

That night I returned home to Catherine's, and because her family were away we had the house to ourselves. As I spoke to her of my day, it became clear to both of us that there was a distinct change in me. It somehow felt like I had left that morning a boy and returned home a man. Through experiencing what I had with my true feelings toward my father, I had been able to contact some previously untouched masculine energy. It was the kind of change that only someone emotionally in tune with me could have noticed, but notice Catherine did.

Up until this point, although Catherine and I had been intimate together, we had never actually made love. It had been her decision to take our time and not rush in, and having mistaken sex for love with Becky, I knew it was a sensible idea. However, being a hot-blooded twenty-year-old male, dating a stunning thirty-one-year-old woman and not making love had been rather challenging at times! Yet, on this transformational Saturday night the waiting ended. Although the details are beyond the scope of this book, suffice to say I felt a spiritual connection with a human being like never before. Becky and I may have had sex, but Catherine was the first woman that I truly made love with.

Before I knew it, summer exams had passed with little drama, a far cry from previous years. I surprised even myself by finishing top of the year. In my opinion, it didn't really reflect well upon the university system that one year's work could be done in ten weeks! Yet, I wasn't complaining. After years of struggling, the changes in my life were becoming undeniable. It was taking incredible amounts of discipline and hard work, but I was slowly climbing back to health and happiness.

However, the time to make some tough decisions was fast arriving. With my final year of university approaching, it would not be long before I entered the real world. How would I choose to live? Would I be able to discover the final part of my cure for ME? More importantly, would I fulfil my desperate decision of three years previously to create the life of my dreams? Even I hadn't dared envision the wonders to come.

CHAPTER 20: LEARNING TO FLY
(SUMMER 2001 TO SPRING 2002)

No man can reveal to you aught but that which already lies half asleep in the dawning of your knowledge.
Kahlil Gibran

As the plane descended toward the island of Tenerife, I felt like an excited child who was going on holiday for the first time. For five years I had battled day in day out with my health; I had faced my worst demons and been to my own personal hell and back; I had lost everything that to me had been important, yet here I was still moving forwards. I looked across my flying angel out of the window at the deep blue sea beneath us and smiled inside. Life really did feel a million miles away from my summers of past. As much as I loved flying, I just couldn't wait for Catherine's and my holiday proper to start. With the stress of university life behind us for four months, we were planning on making the most of our free time!

For the next two weeks, in between sampling the fantastic seafood in the local restaurants and taking long walks in the sun, Catherine showed me some of her favourite places on earth. When we were not exploring the island we lay by the pool, read books, swam, and of course made love together. I had forgotten what it was like to rest just for fun. With my constant drive to create the life of my dreams, I seemed to only stop when my body forced me to. But, for those weeks in Tenerife, Catherine and I just did as little, or as much, as we both pleased, although of course I did still have to devour a certain number of books. By this time my attitude towards learning could only be labelled as an addiction.

Of the books that I absorbed, there was one in particular that blew me away, revolutionising my expectations of what it is possible to achieve in therapy, and our lives as a whole, forever. The book was "Tranceformations" by Richard Bandler and Dr. John Grinder; it had been the only book in my university library on Neuro-Linguistic Programming (NLP), the basis for much of Anthony Robbins's work.

After so many years of life's challenges, I had become very drawn to the idea of working with people in a therapeutic context, and thus my degree in psychology. However, the concept of spending hours on end listening to someone discuss at length all the problems in their life, whilst simultaneously totally ignoring all their positive experiences, seemed rather a depressing way to earn a living. As my degree in psychology was also teaching me (although not its intention), such an approach is ineffective anyway. The fact that 75% of the effects of anti-depressants are replicable with a neutral placebo (an innocuous substance) and close to 100% with an active placebo (a drug that creates physiological changes, but has no bearing on depression) was rather strong evidence to me that psychiatry is an equally struggling field. However, in "Tranceformations," Bandler and Grinder described how studying in depth the best therapists in America, they had created a "super therapy" which had the ability to cut the necessary time for change by an incredible amount. Often, what many therapists took years to do, they were achieving in only a few hours.

One of the original therapists studied by Bandler and Grinder was Milton Erickson, the father of modern hypnotherapy. By utilising his hypnotic techniques they were in many cases able to cut the total time needed for therapy even further, sometimes to less than one hour. Bandler and Grinder explained that much of the reason for their incredible results using hypnotherapy was that most people's problems are unconsciously controlled. For example, a well known stage hypnosis trick is to have someone's arms raise without their conscious control; yet, how could we ever lift our arm with true conscious awareness anyway, it takes one hundred and fifty nine muscles to do so!

To me, the idea of being able to produce trivial tricks such as arm levitation sounded like fun, but the idea of being able to successfully treat life-threatening problems such as eating disorders, cancer, and clinical depression in a few hours, was astounding. Such an approach perfectly matched what I had discovered for myself: change is something that happens in a moment. What is important is how we can effectively get ourselves to such moments of change. With my new understanding of NLP/hypnotherapy, it seemed more and more like the challenge of traditional therapy is that, although generally well-intentioned, it is using the wrong tools for the job, much like trying to paint a room using a spanner!

With regard to the notion of hypnosis, Bandler and Grinder paradoxically claimed that there is no such thing, explaining that we live our entire lives in a hypnotic trance; e.g. talking to ourselves in our heads, creating internal images, remembering events from our pasts, imagining our futures, and so on. The only relevant question, according to them, is what kind of trance we are in; i.e. a positive or a negative trance? They explained that the ultimate job of a hypnotherapist is to break people out of any limiting trances and help them work towards creating the life that they want. As a consequence of the wonders I read about in "Tranceformations," I made a life changing decision that week: I decided that during my coming final year at university I would train in NLP and hypnotherapy.

That week Catherine was also reading a fascinating book, called "Fatigue." After a quick skimming through, it appeared to me to be one of the only good books on the area I had seen. It was written by Xandria Williams, a complementary health practitioner highly trained in many areas, including naturopathy, herbal medicine, homeopathy, and nutrition. She seemed to really understand the complexity of the dis-order, and for this reason I made another decision: to find out where she practised and get her input on my health.

By this time I was past the point of putting myself in the hands of a practitioner and just doing what they said. I no longer took any supplements or followed any instructions without knowing exactly why and without considering my alternatives first; this was to become a highly refined and incredibly valuable skill. I was finally reaching the conclusion that, although many people had more training than I did, no one could ever know me better than myself; I could consequently only ever be the true authority on me. This was a very empowering position to take.

Before we knew it, Catherine and I were back home, her in London, and me dividing my time between her parents and mine. She was using the summer to train as a massage therapist, and I was looking for my first self-found job in five years. I was extremely picky about what I would do, for I valued my time far more than the £4-5 an hour that I was likely to be earning. I figured that I might learn some interesting things working in a health food shop, and therefore walked into the local store and used my communication skills to help them realise the benefits of employing me, despite the fact that they didn't have any part time jobs going.

As hoped, the job turned out to be a very valuable learning opportunity, giving me a first hand experience of one of the world's leading health food companies. Interestingly, most of the staff had no idea what they were actually selling, often recommending things that were far from what people really needed. The expectations of customers were also rather an education for me. Despite being in a health food shop, most people were still operating on the traditional paradigm of thought: they wanted to take a pill and get better; the only difference was they wanted a naturally based one!

127

WHY ME?

Because I was about to embark on the last year of my degree, in addition to working part time I spent much of my summer planning and carrying out my research thesis. As far as I was concerned there was one area of psychology that desperately needed researching: ME. It seemed that I was probably one of the few people who had the inside information to do it properly, and so, regardless of the fact that it would mean far more work than expected of a third year project, I went for it.

I decided to conduct my research in a rather unusual way. Most psychologists (students and professors alike) use statistics, but this seemed to me a ludicrous method for studying something such as ME. To truly capture the experience of sufferers, I realised it would be far more appropriate to conduct in-depth one-on-one interviews, so as to discover sufferers' actual psychological experience. I therefore recruited my subjects from local ME support groups, and after about six weeks of preliminary work I started interviewing.

My findings were, on the whole, of little surprise to me; although of my ten interviews three did particularly stick out in my mind. One involved a middle-aged man who had been suffering from ME for twenty years. Right at the start of his illness his doctor had decided that the real cause of his situation was depression and that any symptoms were imaginary; he was therefore put on various anti-depressants and sent to see a psychiatrist. His wife and family soon took the side of the doctor, believing him to be the expert and his diagnosis final.

After many years of traipsing around various "experts," including staying in a number of mental hospitals for his "depression," my subject was eventually given Electroconvulsive Therapy (ECT), more commonly known as electric shock therapy. To put it bluntly, this basically involves plugging people into the mains, passing dangerously high voltages of electricity through them, and then waiting to see what happens. Due to the massive stress on the brain, people lose their memory temporarily, along with experiencing a number of other rather unpleasant symptoms. In some cases, including that of my subject, the memory doesn't fully return, and what does return, takes years. Consequently, my subject could no longer remember significant periods of his life. From a spiritual perspective, ECT also does serious damage to a person's energy systems and soul. Richard Bandler (co-founder of NLP) has tried on several occasions to electrocute psychiatrists who believed that ECT was beneficial for people.

Interestingly, they all ran very fast in the opposite direction!

After many years of appalling treatment by countless "experts," a counsellor eventually suggested to my subject that he might have ME. Not knowing what ME was, my subject called the local support group to get some information, and subsequently attended a meeting where, for the first time in twenty years, he discovered the true cause of his illness. As he told me about the relief that he had felt in obtaining an accurate diagnosis, he broke down crying. For a long period of time he fought back tears as he continued with his barbaric story, of which perhaps the most appalling part was that when he went to see various doctors with his new diagnosis they refused to accept it, telling him he was a psychiatric case. Thankfully, he was persistent and, finally, one of England's ME "experts" gave him the diagnosis that he had so desperately searched for. Unfortunately, it was twenty years too late; he had already lost everything that mattered to him, including his wife, children, job and, perhaps most importantly, his self-respect.

It seemed unbelievable to me that anyone could have been treated with such gross incompetence; my subject was so clearly just an ill man looking for some understanding and treatment. Although I was certainly not in favour of rebelling against traditional medicine, with cases like this, and so many others that I subsequently heard of, I wondered how anyone could justify things staying as they are? After all, one incompetent physician did not treat this man; he saw dozens of "experts."

The other two subjects that stuck in my mind did so for a very different reason. I include quotes from both of their transcripts:

"When you're that bad...when you're suicidal...there's nothing of you inside...you know you can tune into your higher self, there's a you inside this physical self.... well, there's nothing.... you cease to exist, which is why you can actually go to the extent of getting rid of the physical body, because the rest does not exist...and what that did...I don't recommend it to anybody, but what it did was give me the most marvellous opportunity to rebuild myself...because I completely stripped myself down....OK I did it the wrong way...it's not exactly the healthiest way. Cos when I went to India I had another sense of being stripped mentally. It was a psychological cleansing I went through when I stayed on an Ashram...very powerful. But very subtle, and very safe. But if you are in tune it just happens, and I just remember the letting go, and then the building up, and the, I could see myself going through that again. And so yeah....then I started the gradual process of rebuilding"

"It's like all your masks, all stripped away...like all of them, just the whole thing gone, and just being, rather than anything at all. It's just like, being. I don't know, it's really hard to explain, just being completely stripped away, of all your...I suppose your personality, of what you build up around you...all your little masks, and all of your... pretences and everything, like hats just went with it, everything went. And...I suppose, and then through that realising what you had to start with...realising that you built them all up around you to start with. So just stripping everything down really, to just be able to be, and nothing else"

As these excerpts suggest, as a consequence of their illness both these women essentially experienced a transformation in their identity, resulting in their now living happy and healthy lives. What did they put their transformation down to? They cited the source as trusting the process of life to guide them, and then waking up to their true selves. It seemed that my personal treatment plan was not so personal; I wasn't the only person who was recovering from ME, and I was also not the only one doing it by listening to the messages of the universe.

Towards the end of the summer I had moved my healing forwards in several new ways. In response to Iain suggesting that I consider the role of my immune system in my circumstances, I carried out some research into how this vital aspect of the human organism works and had various blood tests to see whether mine was doing so optimally. I was relieved to discover that all was well. In addition to reinforcing my growing belief that my body was recovering, this also meant that my ME had not caused any longer-term damage.

As well as researching my immune system, soon after returning from Tenerife I had followed through on my decision to become a patient of Xandria Williams. Together Xandria and I created an anti-candida regime for both Catherine (who also had a candida overgrowth) and myself. Although the programme was working far better than that which I had been on with Dr. Mansfield, it was still leading to some serious die-off symptoms. This time I reasoned that I just had to push through; there was no way I was willing to wait the prospected two years for a full recovery. I decided that nine months was the longest I could put up with die-off symptoms for, and so I just kept pushing up the dose as soon as my body was close to being ready, rather than taking breaks in-between as advised. What can I say; I was impatient for my dreams to come true!

After several months of considering different courses, by the end of the summer I had also signed up for a Diploma training in Clinical Hypnotherapy, NLP and Life Coaching. Due to the mass of potential options, I had used my by then usual decision making strategy of turning my attention inward and listening to my heart's guidance. I had been drawn towards a private college where clinical experience was a large focus of the course. This meant that when I graduated I would be in a place where I could set up my own clinic, with insurance and certification. However, before such a dream could come true there were a number of obstacles to overcome.

Firstly, the course was going to cost nearly £2,000 and I had only just managed to restore my finances. Secondly, it was in London for ten weekends over ten months, and I was going to be living in Wales. Finally, I was going to be in the final year of my degree, which meant a seriously intense workload that was already further burdened by my ambitious research project. Yet, as I had proved to myself so many times, if we want something badly enough in life we can make it happen. So, make it happen I did. I sold my car and used the money I had received for my twenty-first birthday for the costs, and arranged to stay with Catherine (who was going to be moving into university accommodation) to solve the accommodation challenge. Regarding my workload, I figured that I would just have to keep a focused mind and prioritise my life.

I dreamed that if I managed to excel in both my courses, at the end of the year I would be able to fulfil several of my dreams: work for myself, earn decent money, and in the process get to fundamentally change people's lives. When I took on a third course early in October, eventually certifying me as a trainer's trainer, many people thought I was insane. However, I was used to this by now. I knew what I wanted and nothing was going to stop me; I realised the value of making short-term sacrifices for long-term gains.

For most days of my final year at university I was at my desk by 7:45 in the morning, and apart from meals and exercise breaks I was still there fourteen hours later, despite often feeling very ill with candida die-off symptoms. I was also working three out of four weekends. Having taught myself speed-reading and mind mapping over the summer, I was reading at twice the average speed, with a much higher retention. Consequently on top of my university commitments I was also devouring an average of three books a week on NLP/hypnotherapy.

Travelling to London to attend the NLP/hypnotherapy course

modules massively assisted in maintaining my inspiration and motivation. The course leader, Phil Parker, made a deep impression on me. He had originally trained as a cranial osteopath, and then postgraduately in hypnotherapy and NLP, and also working as a healer he had a wider view of the picture of healing that many lack. I resolved to learn as much as I could from him and, as usual, knew that my guided decision was the perfect one. I had found someone who was not only an expert in his fields, but also a great human being as well.

As I continued to study intensely, I rapidly gained a reputation for what I could help people do with their brains. Letting people know that I was happy to work for free with anything from major phobias, to confidence issues and stopping smoking, I soon had a steady flow of clients from both university and my yoga class. With my by now constant desire to learn and grow as a person, I was also soon doing lunchtime demonstrations at university. One in particular had a significant impact on those around me.

Knowing that making outrageous claims is a great way to get attention, I proclaimed in front of a group of people that I would help my housemate and good friend, Nadia, lose her infamous love of chocolate in a few minutes. Of course no one believed this was possible, but I made it sound like some good free entertainment, and so, as we walked towards the room where my demonstration was going to take place, a fairly large crowd started to develop. I have to confess that I had actually never done before what I was talking about; I had simply read about the technique in a book and was just looking for someone to experiment with. I did wonder for a few moments if my big mouth had bitten off more than I could chew!

As we all sat down, I added to the drama by waving chocolate in front of Nadia, so as to give everyone a benchmark to measure the change by. The smile on Nadia's face, along with various other non-verbal cues, were obvious to everyone, she was someone that really did love her chocolate! To briefly explain what I did, I took Nadia's brains unconscious representation of chocolate and swapped it for something that she had totally neutral feelings about. Just by using a simple NLP process and some basic hypnotic language, ten minutes later, as promised, Nadia had no desire for chocolate, and waving it in front of her got absolutely no response.

By that evening, Nadia had actually gone hungry rather than let any chocolate pass her lips; the chocolate ice cream had stayed in the fridge after dinner for the first time I could remember. By bedtime, we all knew I had accomplished my goal and it was time to end the fun. I therefore changed Nadia's unconscious representation back as I had promised to. But, something that did stay was my ever-growing love for sharing with others what is truly possible in life.

It seemed that the more books I read, the more clients I saw, and the more demonstrations I did, the more I excelled to ever increasing levels. Throughout my life there had been many things I had had passion for – music, golf, football, and so on; but this was the first time I had ever felt that I had a genuine gift for something. Sure, I was working incredibly hard, and by the following summer I had read over five hundred books in the areas of personal/spiritual/physical development, yet it also seemed that I had an undeniable talent for assisting people in transforming their lives. The more I used it, the stronger it got. It felt incredibly exciting to be discovering my life's calling.

By February, it was time for another surge forwards in my spiritual development. A three times yearly residential group of the Diamond Approach, the spiritual school developed by A. H. Almaas (who had written the books that had blown my mind at the end of my first year at university) was starting in the UK. Catherine decided to join with me, and so, along with sixty other people, we journeyed to Dorset for five days. The structure of the retreat was such that there was group meditation twice a day, followed by work in triads where we took it in turns to dive into our current experience, which essentially meant sharing with two other people exactly what we were thinking and feeling. There were then also three larger group sessions over the five days, as well as us all having a single one-to-one session with one of the four teachers. In my one-to-one session I lost my mind, quite literally!

Ever since that first morning at the hairdressers, I had on an ongoing basis been battling with intense dizziness and bizarre sensations of non-existence. I was also finding that whenever I meditated or dived into my current experience, these feelings would start to strengthen. In my daily meditation at home I would avoid it as much as possible by focusing on my breath, but the spaciousness and accompanying anxiety seemed to constantly be teasing and tormenting me.

As I sat there opposite my teacher, Bob, it started to happen; I started to space out. As usual, my mind and its anxieties immediately kicked in. However, with Bob's gentle guidance, this time I fought against my usual response. I knew that if I wasn't to spend my entire life in fear, I needed to find out what my spaciousness had to teach me; I had spent too long running. But, the more I battled to stay with my feeling of being spaced out, the worse I felt. I was trapped between the urgent anxiety of what I was feeling, and the perhaps more terrifying long-term anxiety of not finding a resolution. I was stuck between a jagged rock and an expanding hard place.

Before long, just breathing started to become immensely difficult. I felt as if an invisible murderer was choking me. My mind was racing so fast that I couldn't even catch what I was thinking; I was just a mass of fear. As my anxiety continued to climax, I desperately wanted to run and scream, to do anything but stay with the horrors I was experiencing in my mind. I honestly felt like I was dying.

Yet, I knew I couldn't run forever. I had already spent too long living as a servant to this feeling. Using all of the courage and discipline that I had developed over the past five and half years of working out my mental muscles with ME, I forced myself to stay conscious. I focused as much as I could on my surroundings, my teacher in front of me, the chair beneath me, and the room around me. As my waves of anxiety climbed higher and higher, I continued to hold on for dear life. Even my countless hours of meditation and inner searching hadn't prepared me for what eventually happened next.

After about fifteen or twenty minutes, the seemingly ever-expanding feelings of space finally started to stabilise and, as they did so, my whole consciousness started to shift and open. While this continued to happen, Bob gently explained to me what I had been running away from for so long: I had been running from my soul. As my mind disbanded, taking my anxieties with it, I started to feel the most incredible depth to my being. I was having a conversation with Bob, answering his questions, except it wasn't me doing so; at least it wasn't me as I took myself to be. I had no idea where the answers to his questions were coming from. I was probably more curious than he was to hear what I said next; it was like I was a spectator in my own body! I also started to feel a deep connection to the entire room around me, as if I was one with everything. It felt like pure bliss. Just by allowing what was waiting inside me along, by contacting what I had been running away from for so many years, I had finally come home.

Before I knew it, my session was over, and I had to go and help one of the organisers count the tuition fees (Catherine and I were helping out in exchange for a reduced fee). As I helped count the money and noticed people around me getting stressed about the fact that the figures weren't balancing, I just remained totally connected to myself and totally in bliss. I had always believed that a spiritual experience such as this would make it more difficult to function in the world. The reality was quite different: I was actually finding life easier! I was living precisely, calmly and with focus.

Alas the depth of my experience was not to last forever, and within a few hours my consciousness had contracted once again. Thankfully, it didn't return to the space it had been in before. Even more importantly, the feelings of space and dizziness I had battled with since I had first got ill no longer had the same hold on me. Having had such a reference for allowing what was there in my experience, being present in the moment started to become so much easier.

Quite amazingly, Catherine had a perhaps more miraculous experience than I did. In one of the group sessions she had also dived into her present experience. Totally beyond even my comprehension at the time, her energy suddenly returned as if it had never gone. One minute she had ME, the next she didn't. If what was as real ME as I had ever seen could disappear in an instant, there was clearly something lacking in even my current wisdom, let alone the beliefs of the medical profession!

Unfortunately, Catherine's extraordinary changes were not to last for more than a week or so. However, we now both had a massive clue about ME that we were not going to forget; we had to get back to the drawing board as far as the origins of our health challenges were concerned. In response to our new understandings, my reading of NLP/hypnotherapy books intensified (if that were possible). And, I didn't know it yet, but finally, after so many years of searching, we were both about to find the answers we so desperately craved. We were at last both about to fly away from our lives of illness. Yet, that was not the only transformation lying around the corner; despite Catherine's and my immense love for each other, our time together as spiritual partners was about to come to a close.

CHAPTER 21: FLYING SOLO (SPRING 2002)

It is a funny thing about life: if you refuse to accept anything but the best you very often get it.
W. Somerset Maugham

Before I knew it, Easter had arrived and it was time to prepare for my finals. For the first time prior to major exams I could remember I actually felt totally calm. I worked with my close friend, Nadia, to share out the topics that needed to be researched, and with my speed reading and mind mapping skills it only took me about three weeks to revise the entire final year of my degree. I also pretended exams were starting four weeks earlier than they were so as to cut out the usual stress, meaning that for several weeks prior I was the only person I knew in Swansea who was lazing around in bed with nothing to do. I even decided to take a break from reading NLP/hypnotherapy books and so took my relaxation to new levels by going to the cinema and reading Harry Potter!

However, things in my love life were less under my control. Catherine and I still loved each other very much, we still had an incredible connection, and we were still best friends, yet the future held something new. One weekend, as was often the case while I was training, I practiced my NLP/hypnotherapy skills with Catherine being my client. In my working with Catherine to help her resolve a long held "issue," we both got more than we bargained for.

Catherine at that time was thirty-two, and although she had been in several committed relationships, she had never really felt her age. For this reason, my being eleven years younger had never been a problem. I had been honest from the start, saying that although I had no idea what the future held, I had no current desire to settle down and start a family. I held the belief that, although in many ways I felt far maturer than my years, being young is about freedom and self-discovery. With my personal journey and evolution accelerating at the speed it was, I knew there was no way that I could honestly guarantee Catherine that in a year or two I would still want to be with her. Therefore, although I felt more love for Catherine than I had ever felt for anyone, and was totally committed to our relationship with absolutely no ideas of seeing anyone else in the short-term, I was unable to offer long-term stability. Up until this point this had been fine with Catherine. As a result of the work we did, something inside her changed. A deep yearning for her own family was awakened, and from that point on the ending of our time together was inevitable.

Flying solo

As the changes inside of Catherine began to emerge over the following weeks, what had been an amazing connection between us, although still amazing, started to take on a new quality. Almost as quickly as we had come together, it became clear to both of us that it was time to end our journey together as lovers. We discussed the future with open hearts and balanced minds, and the decision was made. After sixteen months of a whirlwind romance with the woman of my dreams, I was once again alone.

Both Catherine's and my responses to our break-up were unconventional to say the least. Considering how deeply in love we were, our friends expected us to be broken people as a consequence. The reality was that we both felt incredibly thankful for the time that we had shared together and happily looked forward to a lifelong friendship. It was almost comical to me when I got back to university and told people how I felt and witnessed the shock on their faces. It seems that few people really understood how two people could have so much trust in the process of life.

But, despite my inner trust and knowing that we had made the right decision, I did have some insecurity's about my future. My original plan when finishing university had been to move in with Catherine for a month or two. Once I had set up a clinic, and could afford to, I was then hoping to get my own flat near to her, so that we could be close but still have our own space. That plan was obviously now inappropriate. So, in a couple of months time I was going to go from having paid-for accommodation, student loan cheques, and a very organised life, to having no money and nowhere to live. The only piece of guidance my heart was giving me was that the next step of my journey was going to be in London. In the past such lack of direction would have been enough to create massive anxiety. My response now was very different; I simply put out the message to the universe, "I am going to need some guidance here, give me a sign."

The following Saturday at my NLP/hypnotherapy course, as was always the case, we spent our time learning new processes and experimenting with them. As the day came to a close I asked to speak to Phil in private about how I could continue to utilise the skills I was learning to improve my health. Once Phil had offered some of his usual pearls of wisdom, he went on to ask what my plans were for the coming year. I explained my intention to make a living using what I was learning and to finish work on my book. Phil's response was to change my life forever.

"Well, as you know," Phil spoke, "I've been getting incredibly busy recently and there is just no way that I am going to be able to get to see everyone who wants to see me, especially now there is a television show on my work in the pipeline. What we've done in the past with osteopathy is that we have taken on partners and provided them with a room and clients, and then shared the fee with them. I am thinking of doing the same with hypnotherapy, and I thought you might be the man for the job?"

I was stunned. Did I hear Phil correctly? Was he asking me to work with him?

Phil continued to explain that obviously it might take some time to get off the ground, but if I was up for it, then I had heard correctly, he was offering me a partnership at his clinic. I was totally blown away. As far as I was concerned it was the opportunity of a lifetime. I would have support in getting clients, and I would be working at a prestigious clinic with one of the leading hypnotherapists in the UK. However, more important than any of this: I had my sign, my prayers had been answered!

Within a couple of months, exams had come and gone and, before I knew it, the day for results had arrived. I felt confident that I had done well, but I wondered, how well? Had I done what it took to get a "First"? Had my accelerated learning strategies paid off? Had I achieved the impossible, or had I bitten off more than I could chew with three courses in one year?

Well, it seems that the universe truly does reward a focused mind and an open heart. Not only did I get a "First" (Nadia and I actually got the top two marks in the university), not only did my tutor want me to shorten my research so we could publish it in a top psychology journal, but I had also been awarded the "Best Final Year Student Award" by the British Psychological Society. I was the first student at Swansea ever to receive the award. What can I say? I was reaping my rewards!

However, even more important than my academic achievements and new dream job, Phil and I were about to make something happen that truly meant I was going to spend the rest of my life flying high. We were going to find the final piece in the picture of my health; I was about to reclaim my full energy. Returning to vibrant health was going to mean more than just having vitality; it was also going to mean the end of six years of my inner journey and the start of a new journey. My journey on the outside world, in the larger arena of society, was about to commence. I wondered, was the world ready for me?

CHAPTER 22: FLYING WITHOUT WINGS (SUMMER 2002)

If you can conceive it, you can achieve it.
Napolean Hill

With exams completed and results collected, there was only graduation left before my university years were over. Standing around with my friends and peers, waiting to be awarded our degrees in front of a room of over a thousand people, I think I was the only one who wasn't feeling nervous. I just couldn't wait to be in a place where I would be talking to a group of people this size about how they could change their lives. Yet, whilst settling the nerves of those around me about the life shattering possibility of tripping over their gown when walking out onto the stage, all was not quiet inside of me.

As the organ sang out with the introduction to "Jerusalem," I felt an unexpected wave of deep emotion. This had been a piece of music that had been sung regularly at St. Johns. Whenever I had heard it then it had created an almost unbearable sense of loneliness inside of me, deeply reminding me of the segregation that I felt from my peers as they all sang along in unison. Reflecting upon those years I was awed at how I had managed to keep on going. I had struggled so hard to be accepted, to be someone that was lovable. Yet, having finally turned inwards and listened to my heart, here I was being all that I am. Looking around me I felt the most awesome inner power. "I made this happen," I thought to myself, "I made this happen against all the odds." Such is the power of the human spirit, I smiled inside.

Yet, in the midst of my feelings of power and achievement there was also a horrible emptiness. Whom did I have to share my transformation with? My family, those that I deeply loved, were still lost in their own pain and hopelessness. My mother and stepfather had only just struggled through their most recent encounter with potential divorce; my sister was recovering from major back surgery and was as violent and suicidal as ever. Edging further forwards, tears started to well up in my eyes. Despite all of my achievements, one of the things I yearned for most was still missing.

I knew my family were proud of me and loved me, that wasn't what mattered. I wanted them to be proud of and love themselves. I wanted them to also break free from their lives of pain and hopelessness. For the last four years I had removed myself as much as I could from them, both physically and emotionally, for that was what I had needed for my own healing. But now, having reached a place where I was starting to slow down my inner searching and entering the outside world, I wondered if it would soon be time to also free those that I loved?

Having soon collected my degree and made the journey to my mum and stepfathers, where I was staying for a few weeks until I found accommodation in London, there was still one internal change I was seeking with every ounce of my determined mind; I still had to get back those last units of energy that had been evading my grasp for so long. Although I did have enough energy to now lead an almost normal life, normal was no longer something that I aspired to. The idea of almost normal was even worse. I wanted to wake up in the morning feeling vibrant with energy, to be able to exercise whenever I chose to, to be able to stay up late and get up early. I wanted super health, not almost normal. I also wanted to finish this book. An early draft had been sitting on the hard-drive of my PC for the last two years, waiting to fulfil its purpose in the world. However, before my story was complete, I knew that I had to have made a total recovery. Otherwise, how could I ever have integrity in my claims about the power inside human beings to create health and happiness?

Catherine and I were still close, and after taking several months with little interaction to ease the transition from lovers to friends, we were once again in contact. Catherine had been on Phil's waiting list for several months and had finally got a couple of appointments very close together. I was away on a retreat when she had her sessions, and I therefore had a remarkable shock upon my return. Despite having myself created dramatic changes in people's lives using NLP/ hypnotherapy, it was still amazing to me that someone who had for two years been seriously physically ill could after just two hours of NLP/ hypnotherapy experience such a significant change. That's right, Catherine felt she had found the final key to her path.

Catherine was seriously impressed by what had happened. It was undoubtedly one of the defining moments of her life, and a number of major life changing decisions were the consequence, including her following in my footsteps and doing Phil's course during her third year at university. Now she had regained her full energy, nothing was going to hold her back!

I have to confess that upon hearing about Catherine's final transformation I initially felt rather jealous. I had, after all, spent the last four years intensely searching for the answers to ME, going through all kinds of hell, only to still have what I pursued evade me. Thankfully I quickly got out of my state of jealousy and into a state of insatiable curiosity. If it worked for her, I told myself, then I was damn sure I was going to make it work for me, especially as I was spending the weekend with Phil learning his new process that had been the source of Catherine's changes.

Phil's process was eventually named the "The Lightning Process," and it essentially involved discovering what people are doing which is sabotaging their life (often this is unconscious), using cutting edge NLP principles to break their pattern of doing this, and then using a combination of NLP and life coaching to assist them in creating new life enhancing behaviours.

Knowing that one of the keys to making a major shift is to understand how we are creating our experience, at my first opportunity after the weekend I sat down and did something rather frightening: I delved into my deepest and darkest unconscious processes about my health and my illness. Not censoring and not analysing, I used all my skills developed over four years of intense self-exploration to study what was actually there. What I found took my breath away. It was totally stunning to me to discover that I was still unconsciously running the same anxiety pattern around my health that I had first noticed two years previously.

The pattern was essentially that I would check my body to see how I was feeling, usually finding something that was not right, be it stomach pains, feelings of exhaustion, aching muscles, etc. I would then start to remember all the times in the past when I had been bed-bound and feeling extremely ill, and so imagine similar things happening in the future if I did not rest and be very careful. My unconscious mind was, basically, still obsessed with illness.

Now, clearly to run this mental program consciously and still function effectively in the world would be virtually impossible, for the conscious mind can only attend to seven things (+ or − 2) at any moment in time. However, the unconscious mind can handle up to two million things per second, meaning for it to run a pattern like this would be a walk in the park. With my unconscious mind constantly worrying about being ill, no wonder I was still struggling with my health. After all, thinking about what we don't want guarantees that we get it, for the unconscious mind cannot process negatives. Just like we have to think of the colour red to try not to think about it.

The next time I saw Phil, he and I got to work. We ran "The Lightning Process" on my unconscious pattern, and an hour later I was on my way to a new life. I had hoped since starting work on my book that the final part of my cure would be some dramatic mind blowing experience which I could write pages of stunning material about, totally changing the lives of everyone that read about it forever. However, I have to confess that in many ways (at least to me) this last change was rather un-dramatic. I simply went from running a life-destroying unconscious pattern to running a life-enhancing pattern.

Within a few days I was already sleeping less, exercising more, and had more constant energy. My body took slightly longer to carry out its final repairs than Catherine's did. However, repair it did, and with a few minor adjustments, some on my own and a couple with Phil's help, things in my life began moving to a place they had never been before.

With my experiences in Swansea at an end, it was time for me to find accommodation near to Phil's clinic in Crouch End. Having had bad experiences with sharing accommodation before, and not wanting to live with people whom I didn't know, I decided to live alone. The idea of having no one around, just me, was actually quite scary. However, I also knew that it was exactly what was necessary. I needed to have no distractions, no disturbances, and no one affecting my force. It was time to make my mark on the world, and to do that I knew that I needed to create my own space, a space where I could nourish my own heart and slowly unleash my spirit for all to see.

Having seen a few bed-sits at the frightening cost of over £100 per week, I realised that I would need more space to even fit a desk, a mattress, and still have space to do yoga; this therefore meant a one bedroom flat. However, this also meant that rent was going to be approaching £200 per week, five times what I had been paying in Wales. I had almost no savings (the cost of books over the previous year had got rather insane, a disadvantage of my ever-increasing reading speed) and it was going to take time to get a solid flow of clients. Yet, I had faced my fears before, and I knew it was time to just trust and allow my spirit to make my life happen.

I soon found an ideal flat in a quiet estate in Crouch End; about fifteen minutes' walk from the clinic, and a short bus ride from several tube stations, making me less than thirty minutes from the centre of London. Before I knew it, I had moved in all my belongings and the few pieces of furniture I had (which for the time being didn't even include a bed) and a new chapter of my life was beginning.

The day after I moved my belongings into my new flat, I made the final two-hour journey from my mum and stepfather's house to what was now my new home. After several weeks of searching for accommodation, moving all my things from Swansea to Surrey, and then from Surrey to London, I was pretty sleepy. As I sat on the train and watched the Surrey Hills roll by, I took the opportunity to relax for a few hours. Gazing out of the window, my mind drifted back over the past six years and the incredible changes I had experienced in my life.

As I daydreamed, a curious young man got on the train and sat opposite me. Looking across at him, I began to get that feeling you get when you are sure you know someone, but you just can't put your finger on where from. I racked my brain. My fellow passenger was wearing a business suit, and although he looked smart and relatively successful, he had the usual worn down look of a daily commuter. Unable to contain my curiosity, I had to ask. After all, he lived near to where I grew up, so it seemed feasible I might know him.

"Excuse me, but you look familiar, I'm sure I know you from somewhere. Do you live around here?" I politely asked.

"Oh, erm, yeah, I do as a matter of fact," he hesitantly replied. "I live with a couple of mates in Dorking. How about you?"

"I used to when I was younger. I'm actually just on my way to a new flat in North London," I replied, still wondering how I might know this guy.

"Why are you moving there?" he questioned, obviously feeling obliged to continue the conversation.

"I'm starting work at a clinic," I answered, noticing again the run down look in my fellow traveller's face.

"What do you do?" he asked, mildly curious.

I often wondered how to reply to this question, especially when I was just starting out and struggling myself with coming to terms with having perhaps the most unlikely job for a twenty-two year old possible. Did I go for the conservative approach and say that I worked as a therapist, or go for the honest answer and explain how I helped people to dramatically transform their lives? I decided to go for the truth.

"I work with people to create dramatic changes in their lives, using various cutting-edge psychological technologies," I explained.

"Wow, that sounds fascinating," he responded as his posture changed and he actually looked seriously interested. It wasn't often that a guy my age was actually intrigued by what I did; most thought I was weird at best!

"I would love to do something like that," he continued. "Life often just seems to be so pointless. I work for an investment bank in the City. It's okay; I mean I make pretty good money for my age and I graduated top of my class in Economics and stuff. But, it really doesn't feed my soul, if you know what I mean. I always wanted to be a musician, but it didn't work out. You know how it is. I just do my best and try and get on with things, but this whole life thing can seem pretty meaningless sometimes."

I was genuinely surprised at the honesty of this young man. It wasn't often that someone spoke of their life with such truthfulness. I wasn't sure why, but I felt a serious bond with my fellow traveller; his story was one that I often heard from people, yet there was something different in the way he told it.

"How did you get to do what you do?" he asked. "I guess you were born into a great family, you got lucky?"

I chuckled to myself for a moment, having also heard this a few times before. But then I replied, "Nothing could be further from the truth…"

I'm not sure how many stops later, but before I knew it I had told my story, much as you have read it here.

As I eventually finished and looked at my fellow traveller, I could see tears in his eyes.

"I can't believe you lived through that," was all he said at first. "But you know, as horrific as it must have been, I sometimes wish that life would give me a wake up call. It's so easy to get caught up in the day-to-day stuff, making a living and trying to get by."

I knew he was right.

After a long silence, my fellow traveller continued.

"You know, it's funny but I feel like I know you too, like I've met you somewhere before."

"I know, I'm still trying to work out how we might know each other," I replied, "Look I have to get off in a minute, it's been really interesting talking to you. What's your name?"

"Sandy, Sandy Croft," he replied.

For a moment I couldn't speak. Up until the age of sixteen that had been my name. I had changed my first name to Alex soon after I became ill, and only a few days ago I had finally completed changing my full name by deed poll to Alex Howard (by birth my second and first names, but as a child I had always been known as Sandy). "This can't be a coincidence," I thought to myself, "What is going on?"

Before I had time to think any further, I felt a tap on my shoulder.

"The train terminates here mate." It was the conductor. "You must have fallen asleep."

As I opened my eyes and looked at the seat in front of me there was no one there. The seat was empty. I quickly grabbed my bag and got off the train, making my way to the Victoria Line on the London Underground. As I walked in a daze it slowly dawned on me: Sandy Croft was real, at least as real as anything we can imagine. Sandy Croft was living the life that I would have lived if I had not had an encounter with ME. He was a glimpse of who I could have become if the universe had not given me my wake up call.

Sitting on the underground and looking around at the people surrounding me, the intensity of the changes that my illness had initiated started to hit me. ME hadn't just given me a totally new direction in my life, wisdom far beyond my years, and a career more fulfilling than I had ever dreamed possible. It had fundamentally changed me on a far deeper level. It had led me towards my real self, to who I really am and what I am truly capable of. My encounter with ME had essentially been an encounter with me.

Continuing my journey to my new home, I was filled with an incredible sense of gratitude: gratitude for the process of life for waking me up, for those that assisted in that awakening, and, also, the deepest pride in myself for having the courage to follow my path. My God it had been hard at times. On so many occasions how I had yearned for a "normal" life and to end my incredible uphill struggle against one of the most misunderstood and poorly treated illnesses known in our culture. Yet, I reasoned that perhaps my lack of choice had been a blessing, for it had forced me to find the strength to keep on going.

In the midst of all my pain there was a bizarre phenomenon. A few times I just got so low that I didn't know where to turn, so low that I feared even to cry, in case I couldn't stop. At these really desperate times I could somehow almost sense an older, wiser being, holding my hand, hugging me and telling me that it would be okay, telling me that I would survive and that I had to feel alone for a reason. As the underground train continued to push forwards, I remembered this phenomenon for the first time in several years. I guess that I hadn't needed to be held for a while.

I never saw this being, I only felt him, and I never really understood, until now. There was nothing I would have loved to do more than be there for that boy as he faced his toughest times, to hold his hand and spend some time with him, to hug him when he needed it and protect him from those around him. He probably couldn't have really understood, not when his family were destroying each other when he so desperately needed them to hold him, when he could hardly get out of bed for months on end, or when he wanted to kill himself to end the pain. Yet, it seems he got the message, because here I was moving towards a new life, ready to make my dreams come true. I now knew the meaning of the words self-love at the deepest level. I felt like I was able to be there for myself all of those years ago. It seems we always have someone who can hold us.

As I arrived at my flat on that summer morning, I continued to mull over the life I was now living and the next steps I would take. Having the urge to write, I sat down at my desk in front of me, the only thing that I had put in its place, and began to work on these final chapters you are now reading.

After a while I looked up and took a deep breath. Seeing the piles of boxes in front of me waiting to be opened, I heard my heart to speak to me, "You know Alex, your time has come. It's time to fly."

Maggie: *How do you know?*
Seth: *I have a feeling.*
Maggie: *That's pretty flimsy evidence.*
Seth: *Close your eyes, it's just for a moment. What am I doing?*
Maggie: *You're touching me.*
Seth: *Touch, how do you know?*
Maggie: *Because I feel it.*
Seth: *You should trust that, you don't trust it enough.*
City of Angels

As I settled into my new apartment in Crouch End, I continued to notice the transformations in my life spreading. Things in my family especially started to enter uncharted territory. With George now slowly recovering from her back surgery whilst doing a PhD in English at Cambridge University, she and I started to talk as brother and sister for the first time in twelve years. The changes began with George using me as a resource for information about how to accelerate her physical healing, but we soon entered far more important areas, such as how she could let go of her psychological problems of the past and connect to those she deep down loved.

Having seen the transformation in my life, George started to aspire to create a similar revolution in hers. George's challenges were certainly not mild. The prognosis for recovery from her operation was poor to say the least, the "experts" telling her she would never be able to run again. She was still suffering from manic-depression and aggression towards certain family members, was over a year behind in her doctorate, and massively in debt. Soon George and I were talking on the telephone most days, and she was following my path of rapidly devouring books on health and healing at all levels. I shared with her many of the insights you have read about, and in time, apart from working on herself physically and mentally, she had even started her own private tutoring business to fund paying for her rehabilitation, which included several sessions with Phil to heal her old behavioural issues.

Incredibly, George was not my only family member changing. My mum and stepfather had recently turned to me for guidance on how to save their marriage and create change in their lives. My stepfather sincerely apologised for his treatment of me over recent years, and the consequence was that he and I quickly became good friends. A real turning point for my mum and stepfather was their decision to attend the Anthony Robbins seminar I had been to two years previously. It wasn't so much their walking on fire or learning about human behaviour which was so important, it was more their willingness to take such action. To me it was a clear demonstration that the past was behind us all. Their taking new actions continued after the seminar, with excess drinking rapidly becoming a thing of the past, along with the other issues that had surrounded my childhood.

The consequence of my family's continuing transformation was that for the first time since I had left home for university, I was actually excited about visiting for Christmas. I remember watching the world go by as I drove to collect George from Cambridge on Christmas Eve. I almost had to pinch myself; I was truly looking forward to spending time with her!

After my mum, stepfather and George returned from church on Christmas Day (I chose to use the time for my daily workout) we opened our presents together. It was incredible to feel the love flowing between the four of us. Of all the miracles I had witnessed over recent years, this was perhaps the most rewarding. It was hard to believe this was the same family I had grown up with, the same people who had spent so many years destroying each other through their inner confusion and pain. Witnessing the changes in front of me, I was struck by the wonders of the universe. When I had first started to transform my life I had so desperately attempted to encourage those around me to also do so, but the only result had been my experiencing more pain and frustration. I now understood why; we cannot change anyone apart from ourselves. But, when we truly do change ourselves, often those we care about follow.

My stepfather had bought George a cuddly toy in addition to what he and Mum had bought her together. To me it was somehow a symbol of the future of our family. My stepfather didn't buy it because he had to. He didn't buy it to win approval. He didn't buy it as part of some larger plot. He bought it because he wanted to show George he cared about her. It takes a lot to get me choked up with emotion, but I have to confess I was pretty close to tears. The love in my family was flowing once again and it mattered to me more than I had ever realised. Returning to health and happiness was one thing, but to be able to bring those I loved with me was quite another.

As I continued to share Christmas with my family, I found myself

149

asking inside the same question I had asked at the depths of my despair, "Why is this happening to me?" "Why me?" However, I was now asking with such different meaning. Why was it that I was now living a life I could only have dreamed of a few years previously? I felt like one of the most fortunate people alive.

My family were not the only ones experiencing transformation in their lives. Catherine was also making her dreams come true. For the second and third modules of Phil's NLP/hypnotherapy course I was involved in other trainings, and so not available for my new role as student supervisor. In those two weekends, Catherine had met the man of her dreams in one of her fellow students, and within only a few weeks she and Mark were engaged to be married. As they told me of their incredible news, my mind drifted back to when Catherine and I had gone our separate ways. Despite our relationship actually having been in a very special place, we had somehow known it was time for it to come to a natural close. Catherine had decided she wanted marriage and children, and here she was six months later engaged to be married to a wonderful man who had two kids. All around me the world was full of life's guidance and dreams coming true.

Having spent recent months rebuilding my body with weights, with the arrival of January 2003 I finally felt strong enough to start running again. Therefore, on the first Sunday after New Year, I slipped into my old running shoes and fulfilled one of my biggest ambitions of the last six and a half years. On so many occasions I had dreamed about how it would be to totally recover my physical health, and for me, being able to run with feelings of vibrancy and vitality was the ultimate sign I had done so.

Having jogged to Alexandra Park, I climbed the steep hill in front of Alexandra Palace. It was the first day for a long time with a clear blue sky and the view over London was breathtaking. As I walked along the pinnacle of the hill, waiting for my heart rate to slow again before I ran home, I started to laugh out loud. I knew my laughter wasn't about humour; it was about my body releasing trapped energy. I breathed into what I was feeling.

The masses of people who had created difficulty for me along my path came to mind, those that had thought me insane in my ambitions to change, those that had tormented me as a child, those who had not only lived in judgement and doubt of me, but also of themselves. Unlike the desperate cravings to prove others wrong at their expense I had felt when I was younger, thinking about these people now, I wished they could also understand what my years of illness had taught me. I realised that those who had challenged me had only been the way they had because the pivotal figures in their lives had been unable to give them what they needed as children (i.e. they were in the same situation as me), and that since then they had not found their way out of their past conditioning (of course their pivotal figures had equally lacked the nurturing they needed as children, as had their pivotal figures, and so on). I was deeply thankful that I had begun my journey to free myself and my legacy from such historical entrapment.

Continuing to catch my breath and allowing my heart rate to slow down, something felt deeply profound about my experience. Not really caring that I might look a bit strange to passers by, I stopped walking for a few moments, put my hands in "Namaste" (a yogic prayer position), closed my eyes, and saluted the universe with a prayer of gratitude. I thanked the source of all life for my illness and the gifts it had brought. I knew beyond a shadow of doubt that I had made it. I had cured myself of ME.

By the time I had jogged home twenty-five minutes later, I was looking back on my years of illness and seeking to understand the widest picture possible of what had been the cause. Soaking in a hot bath and listening to the soundtrack to Gladiator (perhaps my favourite piece of music of all time), I considered the three main levels of life: spiritual, physical and psychological.

I reasoned that from a spiritual perspective I had chosen my illness before I was born, as I had my environment, as a way to wake up to my true self and create the opportunity to remove myself from the world and discover who I am. From a physical perspective I still followed Ravi's diagnosis that I had developed a viral infection. As this had spread it seemed logical to me that my body had begun to struggle, and so my endocrine and digestive systems had become severely impaired.

However, what seemed the most important area for me was the psychological element of my illness, and from this perspective there appeared to be two key considerations. Firstly, why I had become ill in the first place. Considering the stress I had been under around exams, it made perfect sense to me that my immune system would have been weak, and so my body unable to deal with the virus that I had become susceptible to. Secondly, and probably the most fundamental element of my years of chronic illness, seemed to me to be the reason I had not recovered as one usually would from a viral infection. Knowing that a prime directive of the unconscious mind is to heal, I realised there had to have been strong reason why I hadn't. I was aware that the traumas I had experienced throughout my childhood had resulted in a severely damaged self-image, along with much inner pain that needed to be processed and healed. Despite the clear paradox of my illness creating more to be ultimately healed, it did also make it possible for me to separate myself from the world and carry out much of the inner healing I needed to.

Yet, the more separated I had become from the world, and the more I had started to consider "The big questions," such as "What is the meaning of life? Why I am here? Who am I?" the more depressed and alone I had become. But, I realised it was also my actually beginning to answer these questions through my thousands of hours spent reading, and in private contemplation and meditation, which had made my recovery possible. Having learnt and understood what it needed to, eventually my unconscious mind had started to once again strive towards health, meaning the various treatment programs I had utilised had finally started to take effect.

What also seemed very important to me was the major anxiety about my health that my illness had led to. As a child I had often felt scared of other people, especially after my numerous experiences of bullying, and with anxiety being a strong family pattern as well, this anxiety had in time become massively magnified by my illness. It was only through Phil's and my final intervention using "The Lightning Process" that I had finally been able to leave these anxieties behind me.

Relaxing in the steaming bath, feeling the hot water soothing my skin, I was staggered by the complexity of the human organism, and realised that it is no wonder doctors and scientists are failing to find a universal cure to ME, along with most other illnesses, physical and psychological. There are simply too many levels involved. I knew that what had worked for me, a combination of a high protein diet to balance my blood sugar levels, an anti-candida and allergy free diet, food combining, thousands of hours of yoga and meditation, and ultimately NLP/hypnotherapy, may well not have been the appropriate combination for someone else.

My trial of numerous different diet plans to attempt to heal my digestive problems had also taught me some important lessons. Although removing my allergens and cutting out sugar and alcohol had made a difference, I had not regained a healthy digestive system until I had learnt to digest life healthily. However, regardless of much of the issue being psychological, it did still seem to me that the typical Western diet has a lot to answer for as far as health problems are concerned.

As with my recovery plan for ME being personal to me, it also appeared reasonable that what works for each person food wise is individual. I had spent over three years as a vegetarian, totally believing it was the best way to live, as so many books on Natural Health proclaimed. Yet, much to my surprise, having recently experimented with eating significantly more protein (about 80 grams a day), including some meat, I had noticed a significant boost in my energy and stamina. It seemed to me that the only way we can truly discover just how much energy and health we can have, is by finding what works for us individually. A quote from Anthony Robbins came to my mind:

Nothing tastes as good as good health feels.

Yet, regardless of there being no universals as far as diet and health are concerned, it was still very clear to me that there were several psychological principles, which I had unconsciously been following, that were the source of my changes. Firstly, I had been willing to do whatever it took. However unusual something appeared, I was always willing to experiment with it. This meant that as a sceptical eighteen year old I was happy to ask questions to crystals on the end of a piece of string, and by the age of twenty I was up for walking on fire.

I was also massively flexible in my approach, meaning I was working on many different levels at once, physical, psychological and spiritual. In addition, I kept on driving forwards, whatever happened. Through more suffering and pain than I could previously have imagined existed, I still kept on pushing to find my cure. If I had given up, I knew there was no way I would have achieved the outcome I did.

With the bath water continuing to embrace me, I also considered the predicament of modern medicine. With drug companies being so incredibly profitable from people being ill, it hardly seemed surprising to me that so many people are dependent upon drugs, regardless of their having such negative effects. For example, the fact that the latest weight-loss "wonder drug," Xenical, only "works" because if you eat fats whilst taking it you get serious diarrhoea, hasn't stopped it generating millions of pounds in profit (the Fenfluramine family of diet pills, popular prior to Xenical, were causing heart lesions in 30% of those taking them and consequently banned. Amphetamines were also banned for weight-loss, back in the 1980's, due to their abuse potential and their causing psychosis).

What did still baffle me was that so many intelligent people are being fooled by ideas such as there being chemicals that cause illness, both physical and mental. For example there are often reports in both the scientific journals and popular media with claims such as "the chemical that causes depression has been found" or "the chemical which causes dyslexia has finally been unearthed." The idea of chemicals causing illness was totally ludicrous to me. Of course there are chemicals that are related, without them we couldn't function, for chemicals are the language of the body (an oversimplified explanation of thinking is that when we have a thought, a chemical is released in our brain). This is similar to a telephone line being the means of making a telephone call. However, would anyone be crazy enough as to suggest that telephone lines make their own calls?

I understood that the reality is that we should not be looking so much at which chemicals are involved in our lack of ease in our body and mind, but what we do consciously, and more importantly unconsciously, that causes the chemicals to be released in the first place. For example, why does one person experience an excitation (increase) of serotonin and epinephrine (the "happy chemicals"), and another person an inhibition (decrease)? Anti-depressants attempt to treat depression by affecting the above chemicals, and apart from doing much damage to the rest of the body, along with actually having virtually no positive impact on mood (see chapter twenty for some shocking statistics on the true effectiveness of anti-depressants), they are based on an extremely limited paradigm of thought.

As I thought about some of the astounding results I had had with clients, I also considered again the incredible money made my drug companies in their mass hypnosis of the Western world regarding the causation of illness. I hoped that at some point I could begin to help break our population out of this destructive trance.

While I worked throughout the day, I continued to focus on what it was that made the difference for me. I thought about how almost everyone alive is facing challenges in their life, be it something simple such as not being happy at work, being overweight, wanting to stop smoking, or perhaps something more serious such as clinical depression or chronic illness. Why was it that despite facing such apparently insurmountable challenges, I had been able to turn things around? I knew I was not born with any more resources than anybody else, and my environment had certainly not been supportive of change. Why had I recovered and transformed my life against all the odds? The answer was so obvious that I realised many people would discard it as being too simple, but I knew the answer was this: I took action. That was it. I had already had a good idea of what to do when Iain had suggested I produce my list of things to do to start my recovery. In time I did make many refined distinctions about health and healing, but they only came from my taking action.

Looking out into the future I couldn't help but smile. I was only too aware of the opportunities my life now held. However, I was also very conscious of the fact that my journey had really only just begun, and that I, like everyone else alive, would still face my challenges. At the same time, I now saw what many people would call "problems" differently; I knew that they are an essential aspect of spiritual growth, and therefore also of life. I'm not saying I was going to start asking for opportunities to grow, but at the same time I no longer felt at the mercy of life like I had done for so many years; I now realised that there is always one thing we have choice in – how we respond to life.

With my book nearly finished, and realising that working with groups of people was where my path was now leading me, I was very excited about having the possibility of designing and running my own seminars. My desire, realised when I had attended Anthony Robbins's seminar, was soon to be actualised. I knew that I had something unique and special to offer, and I couldn't wait to share my ideas with the world.

Getting into bed that night, my mind was pulled back to my last night of health before I had originally got ill. Back then I had felt the happiest I could ever remember being. I had been happy because I was about to start a new band with my friends, because I thought Emily and I were about to sleep together, and because of the prospects held by my summer holidays. My experience was now all so different. I wasn't happy because of the outside events in my life, because I thought I was about to have sex, or because I was on holiday. I was happy because I was me; I was happy because I had the love of my family and friends, and I was happy because I had my health. What a different kind of happiness that was.

Preparing to fall asleep, it came to my mind that when I had been ill, I had so often prayed for the universe to take away my illness and the pain in my life, and all I had heard in reply was a deafening silence. At the time I had thought this had meant the universe was not listening.

I now saw things very differently. I realised that the universe had been listening, it was just that the answer had been "no." There was a larger plan that I hadn't been able to see from my limited perspective of the world. I had to go through the experiences I did as part of my journey in life.

I reflected upon the popularity within the personal development field of "programming our future," a practice I had at times been very drawn to, and considered the limitations within such an approach. Although I knew that goals and targets are important in life, and that often we can achieve whatever we put our minds to, I could at the same time see how this can also pull us away from the plan the universe has for us. I was aware it would be a true challenge for me with my still strong desire to succeed on the outside world as well as the inside world, but I understood that the true happiness in life comes from turning inside and hearing the messages of the universe; rather than telling it what we want, listening to what it asks of us. That is the journey of real courage.

Turning over and falling asleep, I wondered what the universe would ask of me next?

EPILOGUE TO 1ST EDITION (SUMMER 2003)

Even the smallest person can change the course of the future.
The Lord of the Rings

Writing this book has been an extraordinary experience for me. The idea of sharing my journey originally appeared in my mind during the first year I was actively seeking my cure. I somehow felt an incredible connection to those whose stories I shared through their autobiographies; those such as Niro Markoff Asistent, Brandon Bays, Louise Hay and Christopher Reeve. My aim has been to write this book in a similar style. Although in some ways the thought of people knowing the most gruesome details of my darkest moments, my greatest fears and my years of physical and emotional hell is quite frightening, I also know that sharing my story may help others facing challenges in their life. I sincerely hope this has been the case.

I have tried to keep what you have read very much my story, written in my words, only talking of the experiences of my family and those close to me when it has been absolutely necessary. There were some people who read early drafts who tried to persuade me to write in a more "creative" style, and to add more "dirt" about those I love. However, although in some ways these people were more educated in how to write a book than I was, I stuck to my instincts. This is a book about me and my journey, and not an attempt to win writing awards or popular acclaim, and as such it has only felt genuine to share what has come from within me in the direct style that it has come. I have bared every single inch of my own soul, and not held back an ounce of my emotion. I have seen no reason why I should "dish the dirt" on my family to add to the drama.

It would be very easy in reading these pages to cast blame on those around me when I was younger, for my environment was undoubtedly influential in my need for healing. However, such thoughts, apart from being useless, are hurtful not only to others, but also to ourselves. I believe that every person alive does the best they can with the resources and understandings they are in touch with. No one, and I mean no one, does anything without a positive intention, even if that positive intention is based on a misunderstanding. When we judge other people for their mistakes, we inevitably also unconsciously judge ourselves. I actually feel incredible gratitude for my upbringing; it is because of my past that I have the beautiful life I now enjoy. I could not have chosen a better education in life.

I am sincerely grateful for the intentions of all that have been close to me. I know that my grandmother sincerely believed she was doing the right thing by pushing me to perform during my formative years. When I became ill she spent many hours researching treatments and driving me anywhere and everywhere to specialists, which she paid for. It was this help that commenced my journey of healing. Without it I dread to think where I might be now.

My mum has been nothing short of amazing in the production of this book. She has proof read countless drafts, printed off dozens of copies, and sent them all round the country to people who have wished to share my journey. She has supported me one hundred percent in my venture, even though this has involved me sharing many family "secrets." She and I have a beautiful relationship and I have never felt closer to her or had more love for her. One could not ask for a more dedicated mother. My sister and I also now have a very special relationship, and witnessing the changes she is making in her life reinforces my belief that it doesn't matter how major our challenges can appear to be, we always have the power to turn things around when we choose to.

I first started work on my book three years ago, at the end of my first year at university, completing a first draft working evenings and weekends up until late September of that year. At this point my ego jumped on the idea of being a published author, and I worked hard to get my story in print. The reality was that it was not the right time. I soon realised this and got back to my healing path, leaving my book for whatever future purpose it might hold. When I finished university I felt it was time to complete work, and since then I have dedicated every spare minute to doing so. With now being the right time, the words have flowed easily from somewhere deep within me. Almost like a reward for my determination and commitment to share my journey with the world as soon as possible, a publishing deal presented itself effortlessly just as I finished editing. Such is the guidance of life.

My only experience of writing, prior to this book, was of essays and my research project at university. I was always well known for being too impatient to read things through properly, just completing my work as quickly as possible. I had originally written this book in that vein (it was typical to produce first drafts of chapters at the rate of two thousand words an hour), and so the original feedback on the first complete draft was that although I had some great material, a lot of additional editing was still needed. Going through each chapter literally dozens of times since then has been an incredible lesson in patience for me, and I know that it has been worth the extra effort and determination.

The actual writing process has been very healing. On several occasions I had tears in my eyes whilst writing, and countless times I had to leave my desk for a few minutes to get myself together again before I could continue. In many ways it has been like re-experiencing all the emotions again. As I produced each chapter, I worked hard to reconnect with how I felt at the time, often listening to pieces of music that reminded me of what I had experienced. But, now my work is close to completion, I really feel like I can let the past go.

One thing is for sure these days: my experience of the world has been irrevocably transformed. When I was fifteen years old, if you had told me what the next seven years of my life held, I wouldn't have been able to conceive of anything I would have feared more. To spend nearly seven years suffering from a severely debilitating chronic illness, which I was told is incurable (obviously I now know this not to be the case), that many doctors do not even believe in, to face clinical depression and major anxiety, and to be sent on a perilous journey with no one to accompany me, that would have been many of my worst nightmares together. Just losing my health alone would have been too much to even contemplate; sport and activity were my life. Yet, I faced my ultimate fears and I not only survived, I used them to create a totally different quality of life.

I was forced to use the years that most young people use to rebel against society, be it by drinking, taking drugs, or something else, in a very unique way. I believe that this stage of rebellion, although often done in an unhealthy way, is essential to a person's development, for it is how we develop our sense of self as separate from our family system. However, what I had done, as a friend of mine so eloquently put it, was not a rebellion, it was more of a revolution. Rather than rebelling against my family environment and substituting its beliefs and actions with those of my peers and those popularised by the media, I had questioned everything I was taught, everything I was told, and everything that existed in the world around me.

For seven years of searching I put my entire world and belief systems, along with much of my own personality, under the spotlight and questioned intensely. With the perspective of hindsight I can now see why many people found me so threatening to be around during this period, for in questioning the logic and absurdity of my world, I was also questioning their world. However, in doing so I created the ultimate freedom, for I did something that very few people ever take the time to do: I looked at myself and my world and made a conscious choice, asking, "Do I want things to be this way?" In turning inwards, I found my own inner knowing and my own truth.

Included in my many dreams I developed along the way, my heart spoke to me one ultimate dream. I have a dream that everyone on this planet may turn inwards and consider themselves, their lives and our global community as a whole, and in doing so realise how we are creating this world around us, and that we do have the power to create mass change. I hope I may be able to play a part in making this happen, and that this book is one way I can assist this, that each person who shares my story will consider themselves and our world and ask a life-changing question:

Do you truly want things to continue as they are?

I believe the outside world is a mirror of our inside world; perception is projection. Human beings hold onto the idea that if things were different, if life were fairer, if people were nicer to them, then they could be happy. My understanding is that if we want our experience of the world to change, we need to look inside of ourselves rather than without. If we look at the literal meaning of the word "without," i.e. not having, it tells us a lot. The future of this planet depends on what we do with this moment, with the rest of today, with tomorrow and the day after. One of my favourite quotes is something that Gandhi once said:

Be the change you want to see in the world.

This whole world is going to change; whether it changes for what we believe to be the better or worse comes down to us.

Within this need for change, there is one simple thing we can all do that of itself will create miracles. Make one simple decision: to be happy now. Everything we are trying to obtain, be it the perfect relationship, the new home, the new job, the million pounds, whatever it is for you, is it not to be happy? Then why not just be happy now? I believe happiness is a decision we make. I also believe that the more we come from a place of pure happiness, the more the world smiles back at us, and that can also be with material possessions if we so choose, and why not have the best of all worlds?

There seems to be a tradition of desperation and pain in spiritual searching. I certainly know that I myself have been guilty of this. I would study and contemplate life, desperately searching for answers for months at a time. I would withdraw from the world and just think, think, and think some more. If I had the last seven years of my life again, although that is not something I am particularly desperate for, there is one thing I would do very differently: I would make it my priority to find things to laugh at, especially during the really low times; because perhaps then they may be a little less low.

It also says in the traditional books on therapy and personal change that it's a serious business. My personal opinion is that taking our problems too seriously only installs the idea that they are serious problems. Although I take myself and work extremely seriously when necessary, I also believe in having as much fun as possible. If ever you find yourself in my clinic or one of my seminars, be prepared to have a laugh!

If as a consequence of reading about my journey you would like more information on the approaches that changed my life, I would love to hear from you. My highest purpose in writing this book has been to share with others how my world transformed as I started to truly consider my life and journey, and if as a consequence of reading these pages you have decided to in some way do the same, then the countless late nights and weekends I have spent at my computer will have been worth it.

My heart tells me that the next step of my path in life involves running seminars, and that might be one way in which we can continue our journey together. By the time you are reading these pages I will be offering a number of weekend seminars, including, "Pure Happiness," a synthesis of the best of what I have learnt from my studies of the human mind and spirit, and "The Lightning Process," a weekend seminar that Phil and I are putting together to teach the process he designed that was the final step in transforming Catherine's and my health, and which also plays an important role in our clinical work. If you wish to contact me for more information about how you can benefit from these and other seminars, please make my day and use the contact details at the end.

And, finally, the reason that a number of the quotes in this book are from films (rather than just from the more traditional learning materials) is that I believe what touches human beings, whatever our circumstances and whatever our environment, is common to us all, be it humour, love, courage, faith, determination or compassion. So many of us sit and idolise these qualities on our televisions and in our cinemas. If only we could all start living more of them in our own day-to-day lives, using more of who we are and exploring what we really are capable of, this world would be so different. How extraordinary a world would that be to live in?

It could all start with you and me.
So my brothers and sisters,
Be true to yourselves,
You truly are amazing,
In love and warmth,
Alex Howard (Summer 2003)

MY JOURNEY WITH
THE OPTIMUM HEALTH CLINIC

When you read autobiographical books, it's easy to think the writer's story finishes when the book finishes. Of course, in real life things are never that simple. Although my journey with my own recovery from M.E. was over, my journey of life had only just begun. At only twenty-two years old when "WHY ME?" was originally published, like many people in their early twenties, I of course thought I had life pretty sussed. With my self-confidence sky-high, and my life experience perhaps a few miles lower, I entered into a whole new journey: the journey of making my way in the outside world.

The end of the first edition of "WHY ME?" saw me working with Phil Parker, who had trained me in hypnotherapy, NLP and life coaching. He had been a key player in my personal and professional development, and had given me a unique opportunity to work with him at his clinic in Crouch End.

I absolutely loved my new career working as a therapist, and I truly felt I was living a dream that had been so long in the making. To work with people in their time of need, to help create often substantial changes in their lives was, for me, everything I had dreamed it would be. Having been through so much in my own life, I deeply believed in the potential within people to create transformation in their lives, and I think this really came across in my work

I started out doing "general practice," working with issues such as anxiety, panic attacks, phobias, confidence issues, depression, addiction and stopping smoking. Although I understood the theory - having read the hundreds of books I had - getting real experience treating such a broad range of conditions was a very steep learning curve. But, I was more than ready for it, and I loved every minute of the learning and all the extra studying I was still doing outside of consultations.

However, considering my age, it wasn't always easy to gain the respect of patients. When I answered the door to new patients, many thought I was the receptionist as opposed to actually their therapist! The result was that I had to work twice as hard to get any respect, and that was just fine with me. Because, when I did ultimately deliver, people were all the more impressed, and this helped me generate referrals.

After a year of working with Phil, I felt it was time for me to move on. After leaving Phil's clinic, I could now do things in my own way and on my own terms. I was building a dream, and I just wanted to experience everything. The starting point was to set up my own company, and to develop my first audio programmes. The first of these was an audio programme entitled "Healing M.E. The Holistic Way", a series of interviews with four experts on M.E., about specific kinds of treatment, and in fact three of them had themselves recovered from M.E.

There was Don Chisholm (founder of a supplement company called Safe Remedies) on nutrition and M.E., Gill Jacobs (author of several books on M.E. and a trustee of Action for M.E. for over ten years) on candida and M.E., Fiona Agombar (author of Beat Fatigue with Yoga) on yoga and M.E. and Ashok Gupta (who subsequently created The Gupta Programme) on psychology and M.E. With the small profile I was starting to build in the M.E. community through the publication of my book, I managed to sell several hundred sets of the audio programme over the first few months, which established my position in the industry as someone who believed in the integration of treatment, not a 'one treatment fits all approach.'

In addition to my work with M.E., I was also keen to work in other areas to expand my skills and interests. It was at this point that I also started running regular weekend personal development seminars. The main emphasis of the seminars was teaching and inspiring people to create change in their lives. I pulled together what I thought was the very best material I had come across, and put it together in a system that was easy and practical for people to use. At the end of the seminars, I taught delegates how to karate chop a one inch thick piece of wood in half, as a metaphor for breaking through limitations with their new-found sense of confidence. It was a similar concept to the firewalking that Tony Robbins used, but logistically a lot easier to organise.

Changes at work weren't the only ones in my life. It had been around sixteen months since Catherine and I had separated, and apart from a very short fling at the end of University, I hadn't been on a single date since then. I had been so focused on my work, writing the first edition of "WHY ME?" and building my life in London, that there just hadn't been space. But, it was time for things to change.

Meeting someone we really connect with in day-to-day life is hard enough. But, when you are self-employed and work as a therapist, the only people you meet through work are patients and participants on seminars. It seemed I was going to have to think a little outside the box. Internet dating was something that I had always thought only "sad" people would do, and yet I also realised that doing nothing when I knew that I wanted to meet someone was even sadder. So, I put a profile up on an internet dating website and tentatively waited for someone to contact me. I was far too shy to make the first move! About the only e-mail that I did receive, was someone inviting me to a speed-dating event they were organising, with the lure of a free ticket as they were short of men. With this being the only response I had received through intent dating, I thought, "What have I got to lose?"

I only remember one person from that night, because that one person took my breath away, and would continue to do so for years to come. It turned out that she was a friend of the event organiser, who had actually deliberately invited me after reading my profile, to try and set us up. Niki was a chartered accountant who was currently retraining as a clinical nutritionist, personal trainer and yoga teacher (like me, she didn't do things by halves). We had an incredible amount in common. Niki had attended all of Tony Robbins' seminars, had practised yoga and meditation for years, and had read even more personal development and health books than I had (in excess of 1,000). She also had blonde hair, blue eyes, a body to die for, and was beautiful. As you can probably imagine, I was beyond captivated.

A few days later, we had dinner at a restaurant in Piccadilly Circus. The connection between us was incredible. To find someone who was also on such a strong journey of personal and spiritual development was inspirational. Niki was eating only 100% raw food, which she had been doing for over six months, and it had taken her two years to be able to make the transition. I was seriously impressed by her discipline, and it made the evening rather interesting considering I was on a high protein diet at the time, with my meals almost entirely meat-based with a few token vegetables. From the moment Niki got on her train after our dinner, I was counting the hours until I could see her again in a few days' time.

Over the coming months, Niki and I spent every spare minute together. Life was always pretty hectic with both of us developing our careers, but in many ways it was as though we were taking the journey together. As the first edition of "WHY ME?" was published, I rapidly realised that unless I worked very hard promoting it, it would just get lost in the fray of the two thousand books published every week in the UK., so I researched hard to find groups that I might be able to go and give talks to, and arranged a series of talks around the UK.

As I did various talks over the UK, at least one a week, I would fill a backpack with copies of my book and audio programmes and hope to sell enough to cover my travel costs, whilst staying with the organiser overnight if it was too late to get the last train home. As a result of spreading the word through talks, I started to get busier and busier doing private sessions and running weekend seminars. Sometimes I would travel hundreds of miles to speak to only a handful of people, but on another occasion I would speak in London to hundreds of people, and the key thing was that I was getting invaluable experience.

By the Spring of 2003, apart from a short break during which Niki had gone off and done her yoga teacher training and I'd felt the need to throw myself even harder into my work, Niki's and my relationship was going from strength to strength, and we decided to move in together. Up until this point, I'd been living and working in a single room, with a kitchen in one corner, an office area taking up half of the room, and a single bed in the other corner. It finally seemed that I was starting to earn enough money to have a better quality of life, and Niki and I couldn't have been more in love. We found a beautiful two-bedroom apartment in Highgate, North London, and began building our lives together. Not just our personal lives either: by this point, Niki was also starting to treat some of my patients from a nutritional perspective.

With the move, I also had to find somewhere else to see patients, as I had been renting an additional room by the hour in the house where I'd been living. As I put the word out I was looking for somewhere, it turned out a friend of mine had a room in Harley Street which was free a couple of days a week. Although the Central London location was perfect, and the price was surprisingly good, I had big reservations about working in Harley Street.

I was concerned that people would think that by being in Harley Street I was trying to be something I wasn't, and Harley Street doesn't of course have positive associations for everyone. At the same time, I was also aware that there were times when people struggled to take me seriously based on the fact I was still only twenty-three years old. Being in Harley Street would certainly help put an end to that. After a fair bit of deliberation, I decided to go for it.

It was also around this time that we came up with a name for the clinic. After a lot of discussion and playing around with different names, we came up with The Optimum Health Clinic. It perfectly captured what we were really about, as although the majority of people we treated were chronically ill, our goal was not just to get them back to "normal" health, it was to get them to the level of "Optimum Health"

166

that we both enjoyed. We were amazed there was no other clinic already called this, and I quickly registered the company name and websites.

Over the coming months, Niki and I started working more and more closely together, and she started to use my clinic room in Harley Street during lunchtimes, slowly building up her own practice treating patients that I was referring to her. The two days a week, in addition to me also doing a day a week of patients from home in our spare bedroom, soon wasn't enough. A full-time clinic room came up in the same building in Harley Street, which was also big enough for me to run some of my seminars from, so we decided to take it on ourselves. It was hard to believe it, but we really did now have our own clinic, and we were going from strength to strength.

By the end of the year, Niki and I were both exhausted, but also hugely proud of what we were achieving. We needed a holiday, and we decided to spoil ourselves. So, it was off to Thailand we went, my first holiday since Catherine and I had gone to the Canary Islands three and half years before. Whilst we were there, Niki and I also became engaged. I was the happiest I had ever been, and the sky really was the limit.

As we returned from Thailand, I was on a massive high. Work was taking off more and more, and within a few weeks of returning I had seminars in Scotland, Bournemouth and London. I loved the feeling of being on the road and travelling: it made me feel truly alive. Around this time, we also took on our first full-time employee, Simon, who had also been Niki's first ever patient with M.E. He was on the path to recovery, and it was a great stepping stone for him. I also thought it was perfect having someone running the operations side of the business who had himself also had M.E. as it gave him true empathy with patients, and meant he sincerely believed in the vision.

I also started at this point running professional training courses in hypnotherapy, NLP, life coaching and EFT. A number of patients who had recovered were asking me where they could go to train to become a licensed practitioner in these areas and I felt that with my psychology background and experience beyond just the specific subjects of the course, I could create a more in-depth training which would have a very strong focus on developing the clinical skills of the students. I felt that my deep love of learning and pulling together ideas was a key strength in the work we were doing, and whereas it seemed a lot of courses were being run primarily as commercial ventures, my focus was always on how we could develop students to the highest level possible, with the hope that in time some of them may also come and join us in the clinic practitioner team.

I remember on the first day of the training course, sitting there in our clinic in Harley Street, looking out at the students, most of whom were former M.E. patients, and thinking "I can't imagine doing anything better with my life." These people had not only recovered their own health, they were also going to go out there and working with others. I was pulling together my own path of life development and doing something I believed in to the bottom of my soul. Days like this almost never felt like work and I felt like one of the luckiest people alive.

As 2005 continued to develop, the clinic was going from strength to strength. I was booked out three months in advance doing sessions, our mail-order department selling my audio programmes and various supplements we recommended was doing well, and with the professional training course and various personal development courses, I was often teaching up to two weekends a month. However, this did come at a price.

With so many new parts to the clinic growing and developing, and my total immersion in this, there was often not a lot of me left for Niki and our relationship. Whereas I seemed to have a superhuman tolerance for stress, she'd been through it all before in her first career as a chartered accountant, and for her it just wasn't exciting. Although she loved and believed in what we were doing, she also wanted to keep a life outside of work and her decision to retrain as a nutritionist had, in many ways, been a lifestyle choice to have more time for herself, and not to be caught up in her career every hour of the day. And here she was, engaged to someone who had now virtually turned their home into an office.

With the growing size of the business, and not having enough money at this point to rent offices, our lounge had become an office with four desks in it, our spare bedroom had two desks, and we had a sofa bed in our bedroom which we pulled down at night to sleep on. People would visit our flat and ask where we slept, and I'd jokingly reply by saying, "We are The Optimum Health Clinic, we don't need sleep!"

Around this time I also met Anna, who went on to become one of my closest friends, and also in time run the psychology department at the clinic. Anna had also had her own journey of recovery from M.E., in many ways identical to mine, contracting M.E. at a similar age. The

168

synchronicities in our lives were astounding, and she quickly became like a sister to me. Like Niki, her future role in my personal and professional life would make so many seeming impossibilities become possible. You can read about Anna's story at the back of this book, along with an interview with her about the clinic's psychology work with M.E.

After another six months of living under such extreme stress, it became clear that Niki's and my relationship just could not survive the pressure we were under. I was regularly working sixty to eighty hours a week, and to be frank I didn't want to slow down. I loved the constant challenge and excitement of new projects. Niki had been there before, and she just didn't want to live this way, or be in a relationship with someone who did. On one level it was devastating for me that our relationship was falling apart - I loved Niki in a way I had never loved before - yet, just as when Catherine and I had separated, it became clear to both of us that our future did not lie together in an intimate relationship.

For the next year, my life was a fairly consistent existence. I worked incessantly, teaching around three weekend seminars a month, and during the week almost living at a desk until I flopped on the sofa late in the evening to watch a few hours' television and numb my brain. The responsibility of the level of investment I had taken to build the company was also a growing stress for me, as I was still only twenty-five years old. Most people undertaking such a bold venture would have had a proven track record in business, along with personal assets to secure investment against. I had neither of these. I was literally figuring it out as I went along. Failing wasn't an option, but making it work was sometimes incredibly difficult.

Feeling like I had no choice, I just threw myself harder into work, and spent the summer making a DVD documentary about the clinic with Paul Young, a former patient of mine. When Paul was originally brought to see me, suffering with severe M.E., his mother was accompanying him to his appointments, as he was so shy she didn't feel he would get anything coming by himself. He was fifteen years old, virtually housebound with M.E., and struggling to do a few hours' a week of home tuition. He also had major sleep problems, and his immune system was severely compromised, meaning at any one time he always had at least one bug he was trying to get over. Paul was sick and tired of being dragged to see numerous different health experts, including several famous ones that had made him feel significantly worse, and the agreement he had made with his mother was that this would be the last thing they would try; he just wanted to be left alone to rest and try to survive the dreadful life he was now limited to.

The amount of commitment I required from Paul to turn around his situation was immense, and I knew that he would need a compelling enough reason to do so. Something that had been key in my own recovery had been my discovery of my passion for health and psychology, and he needed something similar. It quickly transpired that Paul's passion lay in film making, and I knew this would be a key to his recovery. He started off initially by just going outside for a few minutes and filming something as simple as a butterfly, and that sometimes would exhaust him for the entire day. But that didn't matter; it was starting a key process - the process of life outside of M.E. It wasn't that Paul's passion for film was the answer to M.E., but it was the answer to keeping him inspired to do the massive emotional and nutritional work necessary to recover.

About six months into treatment and working through a great deal of stuff, Paul told me that he now had a real and tangible goal. There was a course in filmmaking at a local college that was starting in a further six months. By the time the course started, he was well enough to start it, and a few months later into the course, he considered himself fully recovered. It was because of changes like this that I loved my role as a therapist so much.

Something Paul and I had discussed several times during Paul's treatment was that maybe one day we would make a documentary together about M.E. Earlier in the year, I had produced a DVD called "Beat Fatigue with Yoga" with Fiona Agombar - author of the book of the same title - and my original yoga teacher Sue Delf as the teachers. I'd invited Paul along to help out on the two days' filming, and in the car on the way back to London, he and I chatted more about the idea of doing a documentary on the clinic. He had in mind that maybe we could do a short ten-minute promotional video about the clinic, but I had rather more grandiose plans in mind. I thought we should make a full-length documentary. Although a little nervous considering he had never made anything longer than ten minutes before, Paul was up for the challenge.

So, we spent the month of August 2006 travelling around the UK making the documentary, "Freedom From M.E.: Journeys to Recovery". We covered over one thousand miles interviewing three patients of the clinic from around the country, and interlinked the interviews with excerpts from Anna, Niki and myself talking about the actual treatments. After a hugely stressful year, it was deeply moving for me to reconnect to what the clinic was really about.

The three patients of the clinic we interviewed, Lindsey, Phill and Alison, had suffered from M.E. for well over twenty years between them, all three of them having been very severely ill. They were all now recovered and having treated two of them personally, and with all three crediting the treatments at the clinic as the source of their recovery, it was a hugely proud experience for me. I remembered that I originally had to home treat Alison because she was so ill. And, Lindsey had originally come to hear me speak several years previously to tell me her illness was incurable, and had only become a patient to prove herself right. I think we were both happy she was wrong.

With the music for the DVD also being provided by a patient of the clinic, and another patient building a new website for us to accompany the DVD, the documentary project had the added benefit of us all pouring our hearts and souls into it. The DVD went on to become a massive success as a free promotional item for all prospective patients of the clinic, and at the time of writing has been seen by thousands of people all over the world.

However, the completion of the documentary was to mark a major turning point for me. The levels of incredible stress that I had become so accustomed to were finally getting the better of me. I'd just got back from a meditation retreat in Wales, where I'd hoped that the time out of London would help me to work through some of my stress and come back more resourceful. On my return to London, the opposite had been true. I was finding it surprisingly hard to adjust to the speed of everything in London. Within a week of being back, I realised that something inside of me was seriously changing and that I was running out of emotional steam.

The eighty hour weeks had now become one hundred hour weeks, and I was running faster and faster trying to drive the company forwards, but I just didn't have enough inner resources left. My physical health was remarkable considering, but I was finding it harder and harder to relax. Even when I didn't have to work, I just couldn't stop thinking about the never-ending pressures on me. More than anything, I wanted to keep the vision of the company I loved so much going, but I also had to start respecting my own sanity. Ironically, in the space of a week, both my mobile phone and laptop - which I seemed to spend my life surgically attached to - crashed. It was in many ways an external reflection of what I was feeling on the inside.

And, to make matters worse, right in the middle of one of the most challenging periods in my life, I was offered a presenting job by the BBC, wherein I would front a television series whilst also doing therapy. On one hand it was like a dream come true, and it would be a massive career break for me, but on the other, I knew in my heart of hearts it just wasn't right. I needed to slow down and prioritise my life, not go from one hundred hour weeks to one hundred and forty hour weeks, which frankly would be impossible anyway.

After a lot of soul searching, I decided to stop seeing face-to-face patients so I could finally focus full time on actually supporting the rapid growth of the clinic, and I also turned down the television series. I just couldn't keep working at the insane rate I had been any longer. I also decided that I valued having more time to myself for a simpler lifestyle, so I moved out of my apartment, got rid of my car, and simplified my life as much as possible.

I decided to move out to live in the countryside, away from the busy-ness of London that just seemed to be feeding my inner state of stress. Although the decision had made sense at the time, I quickly found myself feeling extremely isolated from my friends and support network in London. What was even more frustrating was that the clinic was growing faster than ever at this point - we were getting so many enquiries that sometimes we just didn't know what to do with them. I also greatly missed working with patients, and deep down a part of me really resented the fact that I was now effectively running a company rather than focussing on my great love of working with people.

By the end of the year we had made incredible progress as a clinic. We had recruited and trained an exceptional team of practitioners, had much more robust admin systems, and we all felt we were in a position to deliver the level of service we were committed to. With such rapid growth, and having to constantly learn as we went along, it had been a mammoth task, but we were well on track to becoming one of the world's leading clinics in the area.

But, personally, I felt like a shadow of my former self. Despite having hit my emotional limit fifteen months earlier, I'd had almost no time to stop and just be with myself. My entire life was still totally built around working every hour of the day. Because I was doing the majority of my work running the company by e-mail and telephone, there were whole blocks of days when I hardly left my apartment.

It was in many ways the toughest period of my life, in some ways even harder than my recovery from M.E. had been. I was living in an almost permanent state of stress and overwhelm. I felt like I was trying to climb an insurmountable mountain, and day after day, week after week, month after month, I was driving myself forwards. There were times when I seriously questioned what I was putting myself through, but with the unshakable belief that Anna and Niki had in me, and a determination carved out through years of adversity, I managed to remember the old metaphor that had helped me once before, "It doesn't matter how many times you give up on a marathon, as long as you keep putting one foot in front of the other."

I spent Christmas 2007 in the French Alps with Niki at her sister's holiday house with a group of their friends. I nearly didn't go, so ashamed was I of what I felt I had become. In addition to my ongoing nightmare of stress, my new lifestyle had also led to some rather significant weight gain. Although being tall I carried it fairly well, I'd put on over three stone in the previous six months. It was the only visible sign to the world of the pressure I was under.

But, having been in France a few days, something in me did start to change. I'd spent almost an entire year living as a virtual hermit, by myself often twenty-four hours a day apart from going out to get food from the store I lived above. Being there in the mountains, surrounded by some of the most beautiful landscapes I'd ever seen, there were some glimmers of light. I remember sitting out on the deck, surrounded by the most incredible view of the mountains. There they stood, immovable, unshakeable, and there they'd been for millions of years, as they would continue to be indefinitely. As I allowed myself to feel into what I was truly experiencing, something other than the intense stress I had been so used to feeling started to surface. I felt myself contact the immovable and unshakeable heart of the human soul.

Through all that I had experienced in my life, from my seven years of M.E., to the runaway train I'd felt I was stuck on for the past years, like the immovability of the mountains, there was the immovability of my own soul and spirit. I realised that in the constant state of "doing" I'd been stuck in for too many years, I'd lost my inner connection to myself and the process of life. Something I had worked so hard for in my journey of healing, and was working tirelessly to give to others, was almost completely lost from my day-to-day experience.

The insight wasn't that I could just let go of all of my responsibilities and walk away. This insight was that I needed to also look after myself in addition to the thousands of people I felt I was now responsible for.

I needed to realise I was not superman, and that I had needs like everyone else alive. As I opened up more and more to my close friends about just how unbearable I had been finding it, I found myself more able to share the burden. Not just share the burden with my friends, but to share the burden with spirit. I made a sincere commitment to really start to invest in myself again, rather than letting my entire life be about turning the company around.

Trapped inside me, there was a determination and inner discipline that was monumental, but for too many years now this had been used to keep my focus at work. I realised that in order to move forwards, I needed to direct some of this discipline and determination towards myself. So, I started to meditate again, and I brought to my meditation practice a discipline and focus that had never been there before. For at least an hour a day, every single day, usually very early in the morning, I was there on my meditation stool.

I also started to read again. Reading and seeking to understand what was happening for me at this stage in my own development not only helped my understanding, but it also shifted how I approached my work as a therapist and teacher. I realised that what was happening inside me was a fundamental transformation in myself and how I related to the world. My entire image of how I saw myself and the world was changing. Apart from my awareness of how strong an attachment I had to my self-image as someone who always had the answers and was a strong person, I realised that I also had fairly poor access to my own emotions and the ability to ask for the help of others.

As I could finally start to breathe again, without wishing to sound clichéd, I literally felt like I was being reborn, and in many ways I was. As I regained more of my emotional strength, I got myself back into the gym again in earnest - lifting weights was one of the best ways I'd found to move my emotions and release the immense stress that had been in me over recent years. I was doing a kind of weight training that involved pushing my body to the absolute limits, which really seemed to express what I was feeling. Also, despite having never been much of a runner, running on the treadmill in the gym also seemed to really help.

By the end of 2008, I was feeling stronger in myself than I'd felt in years, and with the benefit of hindsight of the immensely difficult journey I'd been on the past few years, I saw just how much had changed. My focus on developing the clinic had resulted in massive growth and development. The company now had twenty people working in it, including a team of ten of the best practitioners in the UK, and the amount of care we'd spent finding the very best practitioners around was paying off. We were getting over a hundred new enquiries a month, all through word of mouth. This was the kind of reputation that no amount of money could buy.

We'd also moved into a beautiful Head Office and Training Centre in North London. It was the perfect heart of the company, and everyone who worked there loved working in such a supportive and beautiful space. Although we still had the clinic on Harley Street, with so much of our work now being by telephone (due to so many of our patients being initially too ill to travel or based internationally) we were using it less and less. This suited me just fine as, apart from the obvious financial savings meaning we could invest more heavily in research, it also meant I could walk to work to the North London office from my apartment in Highgate, and so avoid the London rush-hour.

The chemistry between Niki, Anna and me was at an all-time high, and I realised the incredible gift we were now able to enjoy. To work with our best friends and do something we deeply believed in was an amazing thing. We seemed to each have found our natural roles in the company, with Niki running the nutrition team, Anna the psychology team, and myself the business side of things. There was, of course, still significant cross-fertilisation, with me still teaching a number of workshops on the psychology side, and Niki and Anna developing integrative models together, which was absolutely key to the integration of treatments that was at the heart of our success.

Just how far we had come was made clear to us in March 2009. We had been short-listed for one of the biggest industry awards, CAM (Complementary and Alternative Medicine) Magazine's "Outstanding Practice Award". I was unable to attend the ceremony because I was teaching a training course, so we decided Niki would go, and Anna and I would meet up with her afterwards. Sitting in the car waiting for Niki to come out and share the outcome, Anna and I were both playing it rather cool, but the truth was we really wanted to win. For me it would be a major acknowledgement of the integrity and vision with which we had approached the clinic. Never once had we sold out or made money the primary motivation. In fact, despite the immense financial pressure we'd been under making treatments affordable to patients, we'd also developed over one hundred audio CDs covering almost anything a patient could need support with, along with creating a vast patient support website of resources that were completely free.

As Anna and I sat outside waiting for Niki to come and share the news, there was no doubt in my mind we had made the right decisions. Our approach was in some ways a lot less 'sexy' to the media than claiming to have a cure, but it was based on our truth. As I answered Niki's call, I held my breath. "We won!" she shouted down the phone, and I sat there in disbelief. If it hadn't been for the huge adrenaline surge rushing through my system, I would have been crying, but there was time for that later. As Niki met us at the car, the three of us started calling all those that had supported us in making our dream come true, before we set off to spend our prize money at a top London restaurant.

As a result of my own inner journey through recent years with the company, I also found myself feeling more and more drawn towards getting involved in charity work. There seemed to be a never-ending divide between the orthodox medical system and more alternative clinics like us, yet I felt it didn't need to be that way. But, with virtually all medical research being funded by pharmaceutical companies, research into approaches such as our own was chronically under-funded. Although I was funding our clinical trials myself, I felt this wasn't enough, so I set up The Optimum Health Clinic Foundation to raise money for and help set up further projects into integrative health.

Realising that there were also a lot of recovered patients of the clinic who wanted to "give something back" and that having some "rites of passage" back to full health would be a great way for patients and staff to celebrate together, we developed the vision of using fundraising events such as firewalking, skydiving and sponsored expeditions. The first ever event was a sponsored firewalk in January 2009, and a group of the clinic's patients were accompanied by my very brave mother.

As I sit here and write, looking back on the past six years of my life since "WHY ME?" was first published, I feel rather humble at these most recent chapters. Sharing so openly and honestly the inner emotions of my life has actually been a lot harder than it was when the first edition came out. I guess that back then I had no kind of profile anyway, and a part of me thought that no one would read the book. These days the majority of people I meet know my original story, and the thought of them knowing the ins and outs of my recent life is a little unsettling.

Yet I'm also a great believer in truth, and by sharing the highs and lows of my life, I hope it can inspire others to believe - as my recovery story from M.E. seemed to - that with heart and determination, almost anything is possible. In many ways my recovery from M.E. was a very personal story, whilst the development of The Optimum Health Clinic has been a more public one, and one that I have shared with my closest friends, the OHC staff, and our large number of patients all over the world. But this is the first time I have spoken in any detail publicly about the immense challenges we've faced to get where we are.

As the public face of The Optimum Health Clinic, I am the one who receives much of the gratitude from those people who have been impacted by our work. However, none of this would have been possible without the incredible team of people that work at the clinic. I can honestly say that without Anna and Niki's vision, passion and world-leading knowledge, I would never be where I am now personally or professionally, and we would never have been able to roll out our mission to so many people all over the world. The clinic's practitioners work unbelievably hard, and just staying up-to-date with the constant research and the developing protocols we are trailblazing is a very tall order.

You might also be interested to read that over half of the clinic's staff (practitioners and admin staff alike) have themselves recovered from M.E. We've been fortunate enough to be able to provide opportunities for ex-patients to get back into the workplace by helping us, and there is no question our systems and materials have greatly benefited from their love and passion.

As I look towards the next chapter of my life, still at the tender age of 29, you may be wondering what I plan on doing next. Well, in addition to the substantial amount of time my involvement with the clinic, Foundation, and various related projects involve, I'm also continuing to develop my work in the personal development area more generally. For me, M.E. is very often a result of years of living in a way that our body can no longer tolerate. It is the result of living in an unsustainable and disconnected way. I personally believe that what we are currently seeing in our economy and climate is the same process. When we constantly live beyond our means and live according to the belief system that the more we have, the more we will be fulfilled and happy, a turning point has to come when it is no longer possible to go on in this way.

People are often surprised to hear me say that I don't believe in positive thinking. I believe that what goes up in a way which is unsupported must come back down again. With the housing market being so over-inflated, for example, it had to crash. The challenge is that most people are unrealistically negative in their thinking, and a shift from negative to realistic appears like positive thinking. Perhaps one of the most interesting questions on both the individual level of our own lives, and the larger level of our planet, is what really creates transformation?

Transformation is on its own a massive subject, and in many ways beyond the scope of the final few paragraphs of this book. However, I would say that very often in life we say we want things to be different, but the question is: "Are we willing to really be different?" Many of us pay lip service to wanting our surroundings to change, other people to change, our health to change, but how willing are we really to commit to being at the heart of this change?

There is a big difference between changing a few behaviours, such as breaking an old habit, and fundamentally shifting inside ourselves how we relate to the world around us. This kind of change very often has to be driven by great pain and suffering, as in the short-term changing is perceived as being more difficult than staying stuck. But, when we reach a threshold that pushes us over the edge and leaves us with the sense of no choice but to make a bigger inner shift, then we can start to allow things to shift. Being able to shift our perception and see our "pain" positively in this way is often a great resource on our path.

Alongside the inner motivation to really look at ourselves and our lives, we also need the belief that it is be possible for us to change. Our self-belief is like any other muscle, the more we work it out, the stronger it becomes. The more we find ourselves in situations we don't know if we can handle, and yet we find a way to do so, the more our belief in ourselves tends to grow.

With the motivation and belief in place, the next thing we need is a strategy to create change. The better the strategy and tools we have, the easier the change will be. But, we also don't want to get stuck in analysis paralysis. Often we don't discover the very best path to move forwards until we allow ourselves to "get it wrong" and try different things. To get moving in our life, we have to take action. I truly believe that in life we either get what we want, or we get a learning experience. Sometimes to get what we really want, we need to have a lot of learning experiences first!

Navigating the paths of inner and outer growth, of finding inner fulfilment, whilst also living a life of value and contribution is not always easy, but I'm not sure it's meant to be. I think many of us have a tendency to seek an "easy life" - a life where we aren't challenged too much or faced with too many difficult situations. But, for those of us who have been to the edge and discovered something new; those of us who have been put in situations we didn't know if we could cope with yet we found a way to not only survive but thrive; we know something else to be true. It is when we are well outside our comfort zone that we discover just what we are truly capable of. When there is nothing left of who we think ourselves to be, then we discover who we really are.

I'm a very strong believer in living life with presence. So many people seem to spend so much of their lives numbing themselves to their experiences through using substances (including excessive use of sugar, caffeine, alcohol, tobacco) to change their emotional state or behaviours that they ensure they don't stay too conscious (working so hard they are too tired to really think, watching excessive amounts of television, staying in toxic and damaging friendships/relationships). The result is that we can quite easily live a kind of life without ever actually being alive. The more we are able to explore the edges of ourselves, get out of our comfort zones, to truly step up to live the life we secretly dream of, the more we discover the innate resources we actually have inside to make things happen.

If I look back on my journey building The Optimum Health Clinic, there are undoubtedly some things I would have done differently. Yet it was my willingness to get out there and make mistakes that meant I learned the lessons I needed to learn in order to ultimately get it right. We can find excuses and reasons why we should stay where we are in life, and I'm not endorsing being irresponsible or foolish, but there is a point where we just have to go for it. Life is about living, not thinking or talking about living. This year, this month, this day, and this moment, will never come again. If there is something we want to change in our lives, now is the time to do it. Not someday. Now.

Whatever happens, however difficult we think it will be, we need to trust that we can handle it. I've seen too many people break free beyond their self-imposed limitations to not only an enriched life, but a life of greater inner freedom, to ever question this. You only know what you are truly capable of by taking the jump and discovering.

EPILOGUE (SUMMER 2009)

As a good example of how my life is these days, I'm sitting writing this on a train travelling back to London, grabbing a few minutes to keep up with my workload. The difference is that these days my work seems to come from a very different place. Feeling like I've achieved so much of what I wanted to, I find myself working because I really want to, not because I have to, or because I feel the need to prove something.

Creating new projects and truly feeling the difference my work can make in the world means so much to me. Having taken a lot of holidays over recent months (I felt the need to compensate for the years of incessant work!), the underlying desire that was there for so many years to get away and just have peace now finally seems rather well fulfilled. This leaves me full of emotional charge and focus for work and new projects, probably the place I feel most happy and alive.

I am very fortunate to enjoy great diversity in my day-to-day life now. I spend a fair bit of time travelling, still give regular workshops and evening talks, teach a number of seminars and on the clinic's training courses, develop and record new audio programmes, work as a presenter for various TV projects, see private patients and am also currently writing my next book, which will be a practical handbook on how to create real transformation in our lives.

When not working, you will generally find me at the gym, on the golf course, on holiday or retreat, meditating, reading or listening to music far too loudly. I seem to have found a good work-life balance these days that suits me. I'll go through periods of very intense work (when I will also be very disciplined with my meditation practice, exercise and nutrition to get the very best out of myself), and other periods of regular holidays and taking time away so I can get clarity on my next projects and what I want to do next.

You might have been wondering in reading these updates where some of those involved in my journey, especially in the original part of this book, are now and what the're up to. Well...

My dear friend and first true love, Catherine, is about to celebrate her sixth wedding anniversary to Mark. They're still two of my best friends and live near Birmingham. After several years of experimenting with various directions, Catherine found herself writing a book on relationships and "Finding true love". I was honoured to be included in giving feedback on the book in the early stages, and I genuinely believe that "22 Boyfriends to Happiness and The Seven Secrets to

Finding True Love" is a beautifully inspirational and very accessible book. You can find out more at her website.

Phil Parker is still developing his work with The Lightning Process. As you will read in the resource section of this book, there are some professional differences in how we view M.E. as an illness. He has preferred to go down the path of using The Lightning Process as a one stop treatment and the only thing necessary for recovery. I did an immense amount of work on myself prior to The Lightning Process, and for me it was one part of a much bigger jigsaw of recovery. This, combined with The Optimum Health Clinic's extensive research, and the experience of treating thousands of patients, leads me to feel very strongly that promoting The Lightning Process as a one-step treatment approach for sufferers is just not accurate.

I am still close to my Uncle Iain. We have worked together on various projects over recent years, such as the DVD "Beat Fatigue with Yoga", which he financed and released through his company Cherry Red. More recently, he has set up an immensely exciting project www.conscious.tv, an internet TV channel with programmes also showing on Satellite TV, based on health, psychology and consciousness.

The channel has attracted some very well-known guests from the field, and Iain conducts many of the interviews himself, in addition to doing a vast amount of work on the project behind the scenes. It is very much a labour of love for him, along with a significant contribution to the development of this area. I am involved in the channel in various ways, including doing some of the interviews and cannot recommend it highly enough as a source of cutting-edge information in the area. The transcripts in the next section of this book were taken from interviews Anna, Niki and I did on the channel. You can see these interviews themselves in the healing section on the website.

I sincerely hope you have enjoyed reading about my journey, and I hope in some way it has inspired you to embrace your own journey with a bit more courage, determination and humour. If you would like to share with me how reading my book has impacted on your life, I would love to hear from you. Please do e-mail me using the contact details given elsewhere in this book.

Additionally, if you would like a free information pack from the clinic (which includes the DVD "Freedom From M.E.: Journeys to Recovery"), or information on our various courses and home study programmes, please do visit our websites. We would love to support you on your own journey of development, whether it is recovery from M.E./C.F.S./Fibromyalgia, or creating the life you really want to live.

In love and warmth,

Alex Howard
London, August 2009

EPILOGUE TO THIRD EDITION

As I sit here at my desk writing this new epilogue, it feels like a very long time ago that I completed the final draft of "WHY ME?" So much has happened in so many areas of my life, both personal and professional. Perhaps this is all another book in the making, but what I can certainly say is that my journey of inner development has most definitely continued.

With renewed energy and health has come a fascinating new dance in the tension between my path of inner development and finding my way in the outside world. It is now ten years since I finished the final draft of the first edition of "WHY ME?", which means that I have now worked longer as a professional in the field of ME/CFS/Fibromyalgia than I experienced as a sufferer. There are many new perspectives that have come from this adventure. What a beautiful, challenging and ultimately transformational journey it has been.

With The Optimum Health Clinic having a dedicated team of twelve practitioners, patients in over 35 countries, and at any one time around 800 people in treatment, it is no small task running it. It consistently takes a lot of focus and passion to navigate the best way forwards, but I enjoy the challenge immensely.

What inspires me these days is tackling the complex problems we now face as a community in the integrative medicine field. We have an NHS facing virtual bankruptcy, with an ageing population and spiralling numbers of people suffering with chronic illnesses, many of which are significantly impacted by the way we choose to live as a society. The traditional approach, despite clearly being a critical part of the picture, is nonetheless not the complete picture. On the other side of the equation, we have various offerings from the Complementary and Alternative Medicine (CAM) area which offer some very promising ideas, especially for chronic illnesses. And yet, in this field there are also serious issues. There is a great lack of regulation, greatly varying quality in training, and also virtually no funding for research. In my opinion the research issue is a particularly serious concern. Without investing in building the evidence base, it is highly unlikely things will ever move forwards in the way they need to.

It was with this recognition of the need for research that in December 2012 I took one of the most difficult decisions of my life. Having privately owned OHC for nearly nine years, it became clear to me that for it to become all that I dreamed to be, it needed a different organisational structure. Several years previously I'd set up our registered charity The Optimum Health Clinic Foundation with the aim of funding research into integrative medicine. But, because I owned OHC privately it meant we were unable to use charity funds to build the evidence base for the effectiveness of our own protocol. Having just had a landmark study published in the British Medical Journal Open demonstrating statistically significant difference in all our treatment groups at three months, I was very clear that the next step was to run a randomised controlled trial in an NHS setting. To do so we needed access to significant fundraising, and the only way to do so was for OHC to become owned by our registered charity.

What made the decision so difficult was the very deep personal attachment I felt to the organisation. For me, in many ways OHC felt like my first child. And yet, in my heart I realised that like all children it had to be freed to its next stage of growth. I had never built OHC with the intention to sell it for a profit, I had built OHC to be the organisation I had so deeply longed for in the years that I had been ill. For it to become so, this was its next step.

In November 2013, OHC and its new charitable structure officially launched its plans for a randomised controlled trial at the House of Lords. It was an emotional day for me. In my speech I reflected back to some of the key events you have read about. My voice slightly choked when I thought about that eighteen year old boy left alone for an evening trying not to look at a knife and considering if his life was worth continuing. Beyond all of the praise and love that was poured on me that day, it was my commitment to the younger me that touched me the most. There is a lot of work still to be done at OHC, and I'm so deeply grateful for the amazing teams I work with who are there day in day out giving all they can for the patient group we work with. It is not always easy work, but every day we know that what we do truly matters.

Outside of my work with OHC, and supporting my own patients, I also enjoy pockets of time these days for several other ventures I am involved with. One that I am particularly excited about is an online TV channel www.conscious2.tv which looks to develop the outstanding work my uncle has done with Conscious TV to my generation. Where Conscious 1 teaches us that we have to abandon daily life to awaken to who we are, I believe the emerging teaching of Conscious 2 is that awakening to our deepest nature happens through the tensions and experience of our daily life. This has been very much my personal journey, and one that I am excited about helping others develop.

In addition to developments in my professional life, my personal life has also changed considerably in recent years. After a number of years of adventures searching for love, I met and fell deeply in love with my soul mate and best friend Tania. As a psychotherapist specialising in adolescents, my friends all agreed Tania was perfectly placed to be my life companion! Tania and I have two beautiful daughters together, Marli and Ariella. In 2012 we were married at Hever Castle in a beautiful and intimate ceremony. My family life is the greatest blessing in my life. Tania has taught me so much about love, family and open heartedness. Every day together is a priceless gift. So easy it is to get lost in the busyness of day-to-day life and, my work life especially can too easily become all-consuming. But, as I sit here now and write these words, reflecting on what I have to say about my life since the second edition was published, it is that which really matters. The finding of love, and creation of family. There is no greater gift.

I also want to say something about what I believe has made all of this possible. Had I not sixteen years ago had my life almost destroyed by M.E., I would not have been forced to that moment where my Uncle so skilfully guided me onto the journey of discovery I was so privileged to go on. Had I not gone on that journey, I would never have found my passion for inner development, and been given the opportunity to create OHC which has been such a huge part of my continued growth. Had I not gone experienced what I have in my professional life, I would also never have become the man I have, which has ultimately made possible the beautiful relationship and family I now enjoy.

And so, is life. In every moment we are trying to make our experiences mean something. We want to label this experience as good, and that experience as bad. We want more of this, and less of that. And, we think we know what our future should hold and what it shouldn't. And yet, what do we really know?

In the years that I was ill, especially the earlier ones, it seemed abundantly clear to me and everyone around me that what was happening was bad. And, so many times in relationships before I met Tania, I was hurt, frustrated and in my heart I was aching because I seemed incapable of finding love or a lasting relationship, and once again, I wanted less of this and more of something I thought would be better. Likewise, so many business situations have looked like one thing at the time, only to be viewed with a whole new perspective years down the line. And so, if I may be as bold to offer you one final lesson in this book, may it be this: You have no idea what your current experiences really mean. Our mind wants to know because it desperately wants to make sense of things. But, the truth is we have no idea. There is a journey we are all on. It is a journey of virtually infinite potential. It is at times heart breaking, at other times we can experience unimaginable joy and beauty. The question is, how much can we open to that journey?

Much is written these days about the law of attraction and manifesting our dreams. I'm rather skeptical about a lot of this. After all, who are we to really know what our greatest potential is? Rarely can we dream a potentiality as magical as the life force that surrounds all of us. That is not to say we don't need to show up in our life, get in the game, and through blood, sweat, and tears, live our life to the maximum. But ultimately, are you in the flow of life, or are you resisting?

I think my greatest lesson to date has been this. Everything in nature is either expanding and growing, or it is contracting and dying. Regardless of physical health in this moment, in the depths of our heart and psyche, are we open to life and playing the game fully, or are we resisting, fighting and holding back? The greatest potential available to all of us is in a sense nothing to do with worldly or material stuff we may or may not have, it is about the openness of our heart and soul to life. That is available to everyone. Right now, in this moment, you have the incredibly precious gift of living. So, why not do it fully? If you are inspired to start an inner journey and have always wondered about meditation. Get started. If you are stuck in your health and you want things to be another way, stop waiting for someone else to change it, and start exploring what you can do. If you are longing for deeper connections in your intimate relationships, dare to show up, dare to be different. There is no time other than the present. Now is all that we have. After all, the present moment is a gift, that is why it is called the present.

In love and warmth,
Alex Howard
London, 2014

RESOURCE
SECTION

RESOURCE SECTION

The purpose of this resource section is not to give you a comprehensive understanding of M.E./C.F.S./Fibromyalgia, that is an entire book in of itself. What we have attempted to do is pull together some of the most useful resources we have released through The Optimum Health Clinic over the past few years, to at least give you some helpful starting points.

The main three sections are:

1. A summary of "M.E. in the 21st Century: You are No Longer a Mystery", a report produced by the clinic in 2008 and updated in 2009. The version of this document referred to in the interviews in section two is the 2008 version, and so you will notice a few differences from the 2009 version which is included in here. The full version of this report is included with the clinic's information pack which you can order at www.FreedomFromME.co.uk or by calling 0845 226 1762

2. Three interviews that were recorded for Conscious TV in the Autumn of 2008. You will find it useful to have read section one first. You can view these interviews for free at www.conscious.tv

3. A seminal article **"Introduction to M.E./C.F.S. and the Integral Approach to Medicine,"** written by Niki Gratrix (former Director of Nutrition at the clinic) and myself in August 2009 (first published in CAM Magazine, September 2009) and which provides an essential overview of our approach to treating M.E. Although relevant to anyone affected by M.E., this article was also written as a "call to action" to other practitioners in the field.

Please also note that whilst I fully accept that there is significant debate over the differences between M.E., C.F.S. and Fibromyalgia, we have not generally distinguished between them in this section. This was a decision taken to keep this section as simple as possible, and whilst I appreciate this will be far from satisfactory for some readers, please understand the spirit with which this decision was taken.

A summary of "M.E. in the 21st Century: You are No Longer a Mystery".

What *is* M.E.?
(According to the current orthodox model)

Do you ever feel that the diagnosis of M.E. is possibly the least informative diagnosis you could possibly be given?

The Fukuda definition of C.F.S (1994), which most researchers use in studies, defines M.E./C.F.S. as 'unexplained, persistent or relapsing fatigue' for six or more months. This of course tells you nothing about __*what is wrong with you*__. Effectively, this is a diagnosis of exclusion when **your doctor can find nothing wrong with you.**

There is no test, no consistent set of symptoms amongst cases, and not even international agreement, on how to classify these symptoms, or even what to call the condition.

The orthodox system sees the human body as a simple physical machine where you need to either fix or replace the parts when they go wrong.....
• The **endocrinologists** have found some limited hormone imbalances, but no genuine hormone disease
• The **immunologists** have found some imbalances, but cannot find a single 'bug' or immune system dysfunction
• The **neurologists** cannot find a specific problem within the nervous system in a large enough population of people with M.E., to provide a diagnostic marker

Much of the problem is, none of these 'specialists' step out of their specific fields to examine the overview of how all the systems in the body may be interacting together to cause dysfunctional symptoms.

__Many alternative therapies fall into the same trap__, claiming for example, that candida, adrenal fatigue, or a state of hyper-anxiety, is the single cause affecting everyone.

The truth is that most approaches are onto at least a __partial truth.__

The problem is, they only have a part of the picture, and yet, they are claiming it to be the whole picture.

Having treated over 5,000 patients in 25 countries with this group of illnesses, at The Optimum Health Clinic we *know* that **M.E. is a process where __multiple systems__, both psychological and physical, are __interacting together__ in a dysfunctional way, resulting in the various symptoms experienced.**

190

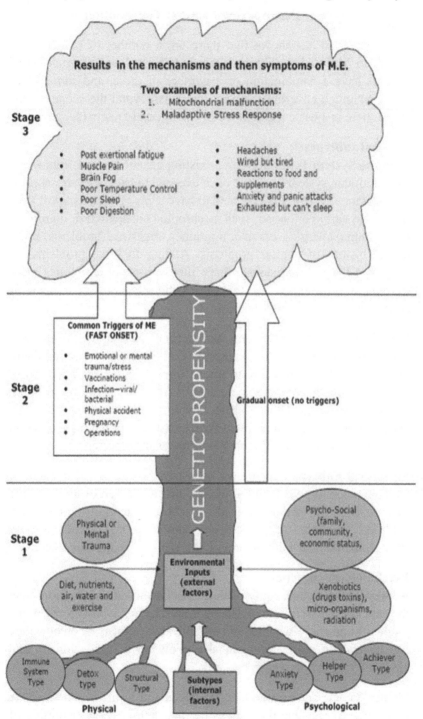

Stage 1: Predisposing Factors: The 7 Subtypes

Our experience has shown that there are a number of predisposing factors to M.E./C.F.S./Fibromyalgia, but internal and external. Most patients have a combination of a number of these, and some all of them. Although covering these in details is beyond the scope of this report, here is a basic explanation of the internal factors (subtypes)

Physical subtypes:
Immune System Types: have pre-existing genetics or constitutionally weak immune systems, or have been exposed to excessive stressors on their immune system. Patients tend to have signs of digestive problems right from early childhood, such as chronic constipation or diarrhoea, IBS, asthma, allergies, eczema, migraines, menstrual problems, and a family history of similar problems. Adding to these problems, or triggering them, are amongst others, the over-use of antibiotics, non-steroidal anti-inflammatory drugs, parasitic infections, operations, or certain viral or bacterial infections.

Detox Types: have problems with toxins, caused by pre-existing genetic or constitutional weaknesses at detoxifying or tolerating them, or have had major exposure to toxins through either their work or a specific event. Early signs include sensitivity to chemicals in paint, petrol or perfumes. Other risk factors can include mercury fillings, vaccinations, living in a polluted area, pesticides, or having worked in a building where 'sick building syndrome' was suspected.

Structural Subtypes: may have been born with a spinal imbalance, which has led to poor lymph drainage, and a back-up of toxins in the system. Once ill, patients can also become structurally imbalanced, leading to these detoxification complications. Patients with temporomandibular joint disorder (TMD) also fall into this category.

Psychological subtypes:
Achiever Types: constantly push themselves to do and be more than they are currently capable of. Characterised by an inability to 'be in the moment', and enjoy 'what is', and instead, always focusing on how they can be and do more. This can also show up as perfectionism and always trying to 'get it right'.

Helper Types: constantly place the needs and wants of others above their own. They value themselves by their helping and supporting of others, and although in the eyes of society might be perceived as a 'good person', are often actually giving from a place of inner lacking and neediness.

Anxiety Types: have an internal sense of fear, danger, and threat. They deal with this either by being an outwardly fearful type, or by becoming the opposite, and constantly try to convince themselves and others they are not afraid. Under the surface is an ongoing sense of things 'not being OK' and the world not being able to support them.

Trauma Types: trauma can either be a major event such as a natural disaster, or some kind of physical, mental, emotional or sexual abuse, or what is known as 'Developmental Trauma' where there is no single event, but happens to someone who has grown up in an 'unheld and unsupported environment' - these kinds of trauma are not generally digested without professional assistance, and therefore take a long term toll on the body when not healthily worked through.

Stage 2: Triggers

This explains the factors that predispose us to developing M.E., although for many of us these were already there - so <u>why did we develop M.E. when we did?</u>

Fast Onset:
With these predisposing factors, it then takes a trigger to push us into M.E. This is sort of like 'the final straw that breaks the camel's back'.

Examples include:
- Severe emotional or mental distress - including divorce, loss of a loved one
- Vaccinations
- Infection - viral or bacterial

Gradual Onset:
Sometimes there is no 'final straw' but a gradual emergence of symptoms. This is the result of too many of the subtypes being out of balance for too long.

Predisposing factors (the subtypes), followed by a trigger (or not if a gradual onset), finally results in M.E.

Stage 3: The Resultant Symptoms
What symptoms you develop depends upon:
1. Your genes (although the research suggests that genetics play a relatively small role in M.E./C.F.S./Fibromyalgia)
2. What stage of the illness you are at
3. What your predisposing factors were

As explained earlier, every case of M.E. is different, and there are many 'mechanisms' that actually explain the symptoms people experience. In this basic outline we are going to focus on just a few of those. And yet, these two factors alone can explain a great number of the symptoms experienced by many patients.

MITOCHONDRIAL MALFUNCTION... JUST ONE EXAMPLE

Your mitochondria are effectively the <u>powerhouses of your cells</u>, and therefore responsible for your <u>energy production at a cellular level</u>.

They are the equivalent of the engine in a car. If you've ever wondered what on earth is actually causing so many people to feel fatigued, here is your answer:

You have **50 trillion or so cells in your body**, and nearly all of them have a little part in them called 'mitochondria'.

Energy in your body is called A.T.P. (adenosine triphosphate), and is similar to a car engine - A.T.P. is continually recycled (from A.D.P. in the mitochondria). When this cycle of recycling is going too slowly, your energy is rationed. When your A.T.P. is gone, this is similar to the experience of someone 'pulling the plug' - your body can't make A.T.P. from scratch, and this is why it can take days or even weeks to recover from a 'crash.'

What is particularly interesting about this for patients is that it explains why they can be fine doing a particular activity, fine even the day after, and then suddenly, 'out of nowhere', they 'crash'; it is at this point that the A.T.P runs out - prior to this, there is often a day or so of feeling 'hyper' and unable to relax.

The key to treating this is in the understanding of what is blocking A.T.P production, and giving the body the support it needs to rebuild its' reserves. By testing your A.T.P. production, we can basically measure (on a cellular level), your body's ability to produce energy.

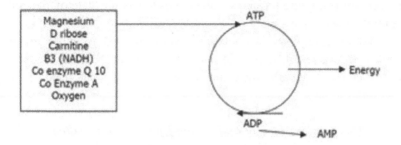

We can then treat this directly, by supporting your body in correcting the underlying imbalances.

Some other examples of physical imbalances:
- Thyroid and adrenal imbalances
- Digestive imbalances - such as parasites, Candida, Dysbiosis, leaky gut, malabsorption
- Growth and sex hormone imbalances
- Allergies/Food intolerances
- Fibromyalgia and Multiple Chemical Sensitivity
- Metabolic Typing and blood sugar imbalances
- Metal or pesticide toxicity
- Mitochondrial malfunction
- Immune system dysfunction (chronic viral, bacterial infections and TH2 dominance)
- Low glutathione and methylation cycle blocks
- Lymph and liver detoxification problems
- Nervous system and neurotransmitter imbalances (insomnia/ anxiety
  etc)
- Other specific problems such as PMS and migraines

MALADAPTIVE STRESS RESPONSE

The maladaptive stress response is the state of 'high alert' the body often goes into <u>in reaction</u> to experiencing an illness such as M.E.

Having stressors prior to developing the illness often also play a role, but the actual experience of M.E. is a major trauma in itself. For example, not knowing what is wrong, why it is wrong, will you ever recover, are you going to relapse, all creates a massive state of 'danger' within the nervous system.

As far as your body is concerned, your survival is under major threat, and as a result, it goes into a state of "Fight, flight or freeze," even when this is actually the exact opposite state the body needs to be in, in order to heal.

This failure to adapt and normalise* *is why it is called* *the maladaptive stress response.

There are *very real physical effects* of being in this state:

- Digestive system - inability to absorb nutrients from food
- Immune system - adverse reaction to supplements
- Nervous system - 'tired but wired'- exhausted all day but unable to sleep at night

Several therapies over recent years have become popular for treating M.E. from a psychological perspective, and look at different aspects of the Maladaptive Stress Response:

Reverse Therapy works with the theory that the patient must listen to the 'Bodymind' (the emotions and body messages). However, it ignores the fact that many patients are in a strong anxiety state, which makes the messages they receive both unclear and confused.

The Lightning Process addresses the anxiety state, but fails to take into account the underlying tendencies (The Helper and Achiever subtypes). It tends to encourage patients to push themselves where this may not be appropriate, without dealing with the underlying subtypes which were instrumental in causing them to become ill in the first place. The result is that a subgroup of patients do feel better for a while, but then often go on to relapse.

The trouble is that such approaches are only partial in their understanding, and as a result can actually in some cases be quite damaging, by further adding to the confusion and frustration already being felt by patients.

In reality, you need to treat the subtype causes, ***and*** *the Maladaptive Stress Response reaction.*

Healing M.E., C.F.S. and Fibromyalgia in the 21st Century

Healing M.E., C.F.S. and Fibromyalgia in the 21st Century
Iain McNay interviews Alex Howard

Iain: Hello, and welcome to Conscious TV. My name is Iain McNay and today we're going to talk about M.E., also known as Chronic Fatigue Syndrome, and we're going to have an overview of the subject by Alex Howard. Hi Alex.

Alex: Hi.

I: Alex was diagnosed with M.E when he was fifteen years old, and suffered for nearly seven years. He wrote a book as an account of his experiences - of how he got M.E., how he dealt with it and how in the end he actually recovered from M.E. So, Alex, let's move straight onto an overview. You did a report that you called "M.E. in the 21st Century - You are no longer a mystery", which I liked, because I think that's what many people with M.E. think. They actually think they're a mysterious case and Doctors can't actually do anything to cure them, and that's obviously not true.

A: Yes, well as you mentioned, I had M.E. myself for seven years, and was first diagnosed in the mid 90's. Back at that point, you'd go to your Doctor with tiredness and dizziness and those kinds of symptoms, and there really was no answer. So I went down a path of trying a number of different alternative therapies and nutrition-based therapies and really just doing everything I could to try and turn around what was obviously a very difficult situation. I spent the first two years virtually bed-bound, hardly able to do anything, and I really got to the point where I just could not continue with life that way, a point where I saw that my life was going to go in one of two directions: I was going to either continue waiting for the medical system to have some kind of answers, or I was going to have to do something more proactive myself to turn the situation around.

What really started out as a desperate search for myself, went on to become a clinic that now works with quite a number of people. Even now for a lot of people diagnosed with M.E., chronic fatigue, or fibromyalgia, as a kind of whole group of illnesses (that maybe we'll talk a bit about in this interview), I think one of the really difficult things is that you may have that label but it doesn't really tell you what's actually wrong with you. And that was very difficult, especially in the early days of an illness that affects a lot more people now. You have this label, but it doesn't actually tell you what's actually going on inside of your body.

I: OK, so somebody doesn't feel well in this ongoing situation, they go to their Doctor and the Doctor says you've got M.E., where do they go from there?

A: Well, there are treatments that are available on the NHS in the UK, and in America there are similar kinds of things that are available, but they really involve managing symptoms rather than actually understanding the underlying things that are going on.

I: And the symptoms, so we're clear, are that the person is very tired, can have muscle pains and so on....

A: Yes. This in itself brings up a big challenge in this area, in that the symptoms are different in different people. Some people just have fatigue, and they don't really have much apart from that, but they're just really struggling to keep up with a day to day life. That's at one level. At the other extreme you have people who have fatigue, but can also have headaches, dizziness, light-and-sound-sensitivity, muscle pains - a whole range of other things that can be going on; and it can range from people who are literally in a darkened room, who are so ill they're unable to do anything (even get out of bed), to people who can pretty much keep up with life, but there's not the energy that should really be there, and they're more susceptible to either viruses or colds and they get knocked out more than other people would. So you've got a whole range of different people with different symptoms and different expressions of what's going on. Then you have a Western model of needing to classify people into one group, with one list of symptoms, to then go and look for one treatment that's going to work for all of those people. One of the things that we say at the clinic is that M.E. is not an illness in the traditional sense; it is really a process of a number of things in the body that have gone out of balance.

I: So it's interesting you say that things have gone out of balance in the body. What do you mean by that?

A: Well the body's got a whole bunch of different systems, from the immune system to the digestive system, to the endocrine system and as I was saying in the medical model, it's always looking for one thing that you can give a drug or a treatment for, but in the way that we work with M.E., we are looking at different stages of the illness. We also, for example, look at certain predisposing factors, i.e. things that could be going on prior to becoming ill that can predispose someone towards something like M.E. or chronic fatigue.

I: So what's an example of that maybe?

A: So, we classify pre-disposing factors on the Psychology side and the Nutrition side. On the psychology side, there are what are called energy-depleting psychologies - so ways of approaching our self or the world, which are burning up more resources than will be helpful. So an example would be what we call "The Achiever Subtype," and these are people who are always pushing themselves and driving themselves to do and to be more than they currently are, and you can imagine that if someone is living in that way consistently, it becomes very depleting to the system.

I: So what you're saying is their resources are finite and they only last so long and then resources start to diminish and they can't do the same thing anymore that they were doing and want to do?

A: Yes. And of course what most people do faced with a situation where they're used to pushing themselves, and the resources start to diminish, is they just push themselves harder.

I: That's even worse.

A: That's their default system. It's their way of approaching life. Other examples on the psychology side would be "The Helper Subtype," and these are people who are always looking to help other people and put other people's needs as higher than their own, and if someone does that for long enough after a while that becomes depleting. On the psychology side we also refer to an "Anxiety Subtype," and this is where people have more of a sense of ongoing background worry and anxiety in maybe a situation that somebody else would be able to let go of more easily, but it kind of nags and it's kind of there and they're carrying it more.

We also refer to a "Trauma Subtype," and this is where someone's got some kind of trauma in the past which has never been properly released or worked through. So, if we look at these kinds of subtypes on the psychology side, these are all things which place demands upon our systems in ways that other people may not experience. Now of course there are people out there that have these subtypes that don't get M.E., it's just one component.

I: I think, if I can just interrupt you there, it's one of the difficult things for people, because they're with their friends and they're not doing anything different from their friends and they're getting sick and their friends are okay.

A: Yes, and we'll come to in a little bit how although we have these predisposing factors, we still require triggers and things to cause M.E. or chronic fatigue to manifest. Before we come to that though, we also refer to certain subtypes on the physical side. We talk about an "Immune Subtype;" and this is where people from a very young age were more likely to catch colds and viruses and they just seemed to be getting sick a lot, so there's a weakness in the immune system.

We also talk about a "Detox Subtype," and this is where people seem to throughout their life have had issues around toxicity, because they've been overexposed to chemicals or organophosphates and those kinds of things, and maybe they've got food intolerances, but you can see they have trouble with detoxifying substances that maybe other people will be okay with. And just a final of these seven subtypes as we classify them, is what we call the "Diet and Lifestyle Type." This is where people (and I think that it's obviously becoming more and more prevalent in the western world), just don't look after themselves. You know, lots of drinking, smoking, partying, not resting, and living life in a way that's placing too many demands on themselves. Shift work is a great example of that, people that are up five to six nights a week working and they're constantly pulling their body out of its natural balance and ways of being.

So you have either one, a few, or a collection of these predisposing factors (subtypes) which are there, but as you mentioned lots of people in society can have those things going on without it necessarily manifesting as something like M.E. A couple of things about that, firstly these ideas are embryonic in that they're based on clinical experience rather than scientific research studies, but we believe there's a genetic component which may well be going on. For example, why does one person have all of these predisposing factors and develop M.E. and someone else develops maybe cancer or heart disease or something else? But, there's normally a trigger event of something that happens that with all of these predisposing factors weakening the system, pushes them into some kind of burnout. That can be anything from a very stressful life event, like the loss of a job, or loss of a loved one, or divorce, or something like that, to being exposed to some kind of virus (glandular fever is a common example).

There are also many people who have what we call gradual onset, where it's the predisposing factors, with so much out of balance, over so much time, that the body simply cannot keep going. I think a really helpful way to look at it is M.E. is really an example of when the demands being placed upon the system are more than the system can handle and when it's for long enough, something snaps.

I: The more you talk about it, the more I realise this is a lot of information, and for someone who doesn't know about health and just wants to live their life, especially a young person, this is quite daunting. That they've got to be aware of this, they've got to make sure they don't overstretch themselves doing this particular sport they want to do, or their studying for examinations and their social life's imbalanced, that they don't have too much binge drinking and all the rest of it, and that's a lot for a young person to take on board.

A: And as I was saying, it's where the demands are placed upon the system for long enough, and then it's like a fuse going. To give you some statistics for example, it's believed there are around _ million people in the UK that are affected with M.E. severe enough that it's been diagnosed. My sense is that it's probably a lot higher than that. They are quite old statistics and I think a lot of people are affected with symptoms, who aren't going to their doctors...

I: And most people are tired! I get tired you know....

A: It's an interesting point, because if you think about it as being a line where you've got at one end people that are just a bit more tired than maybe they used to be, and at the other end people who are severely affected and housebound or bed-bound with M.E. as an illness, you see that, there is a vast range of different people with different levels of impairment. Most people don't have as much energy as they might have, but also most people live fairly stressful lives in the western world. The human body adjusts quite slowly genetically over time to become used to the environment we're in, and if we look at the changes

202

in our environment in even the past ten years they are major. Back in 1996 when I first got ill mobile phones and the internet had only just started to gain mass appeal, and now you're out for a walk relaxing and your phone's ringing the whole time. It wasn't like that even ten years ago.

So, a lot has changed in our environment and M.E. is an example of it being too much for people to handle, and a useful analogy that people have used is it's a bit like down in the mines, they would take a canary down because a canary would get affected by the poisonous gases much more quickly than anybody else would, and that would act as a warning. In some ways people with M.E. are like the canaries, they are the warnings that the way that we're living for a lot of people is placing too many demands...

I: It's funny you should mention that, I was reading about that the other day and I read what happened originally was the canary would go unconscious but they didn't let the canary die, they would take the canary out and they would all leave straight away, and so they'd catch it at a point before the canary died, and that's intelligence!

A: Yes, that's not what generally happens in the western world.

I: Absolutely.

A: And, as we mentioned before as well, what often happens is as people start to get ill, they often will continue to do the things which caused them to get ill in the first place. As a clinic we've treated thousands of people and I've been responsible for seeing a lot of different M.E. cases, and you'd be amazed by the number of people that will say things like, "I started to develop symptoms and I was really struggling to get through the day at work and I thought that I was just unfit! Or I thought I was just being lazy, so I went and joined the gym!"
I: That probably isn't a very good idea!

A: Well statistically, with M.E. one of the things that's been found is early diagnosis is a strong indicator of a good prognosis going forwards, because it means we stop doing the things which are constantly weakening and damaging the system.

I: Yes, but we also have to listen and we have to be willing to go along with the advice we are given, which isn't easy. You get a bit down energy wise and you adjust things a little bit and you feel a bit better and you start really trying to race up to back to where you were. It's very hard, that mental discipline.

A: It is, and there's so much conflicting advice as well, you know a lot of people that we've been responsible for treating, when they first went to their doctor were told, "Oh, you're just depressed" or "What are you complaining about?", and so the culture we live in kind of supports ignoring how we feel to keep up with the status quo and what we're used to doing. A key lesson for a lot of people in their recovery is actually to stop trying to hold on to their life, and actually have an acceptance of what's happening. And when I say acceptance, I don't mean giving in and saying "This is my life, I'm never going to get better from this," but actually creating an environment which is going to be supportive to recovery, and that can involve some very difficult life decisions sometimes.

I: Yes, and is everybody equipped to do that?

A: Well, I think people often don't realise what they are capable of until they have no choice. Also, as we mentioned there's so much conflicting advice. If you have an injury like a broken arm or leg and people can see it, you go into work and people will often help you and it's a very visible thing. With M.E. it's treated with a lot of scepticism by most people. People will say I've got chronic fatigue or M.E. and people will often say to them "Well, I think I've got that too, I'm tired all the time." and they don't quite understand that there's a difference between someone that can't get through a day without having to go to bed nd the many people who do just have a certain amount of fatigue.

So people meet with so much scepticism and so much lack of understanding in the world around them, and in that environment it's very difficult for people to be accepting of themselves and what's happening. You know when I got ill when I was fifteen up until that point I'd been very into sport, very active and I defined myself a lot by being that way. To go from that to then struggling to get through a day at school and not being able to do P.E. lessons and instead have to go home and rest when all my friends would go and play football, was very difficult to explain to people.

I: Yes, and also psychologically you have to take that on board yourself and that is not easy.

A: Absolutely. So, moving on, we have talked about predisposing factors and triggers, and there's a whole other section which is often very key with M.E., which is the perpetuating factors. We don't want to get too complex here in that there are a lot of different parts to look at, but just a couple of components I think are really important. One of which is, if there's been stress prior to being ill, when somebody gets ill, there's a massive new stress, and that's the stress of being ill, especially so with an illness where it feels like no-one can really tell you what's wrong with you and people are often questioning you, thinking you're being lazy and you need to just get on with it. Often life was stressful before, and you've still got all the same demands, but you've got no capacity to meet those demands. That's incredibly stressful for people to deal with, and then you've got kind of the repeating questions inside of the mind of "What's wrong with me? Why is it wrong with me? Will I ever get better? What shall I do? Shall I rest? Shall I push myself?" and all this stuff's going on in the background and of course that drives up the nervous system.

And when the nervous system drives up in that way, we're in exactly the opposite state to do what we need to do, to be able to recover and heal. To put it in the simplest terms possible, your body can either be in a stress state, or it can be in a healing state, and if you're in a stress state, you're using more energy than you're building. When I say build energy, I mean through eating food and rest and those kinds of things. If you're in a healing state, you're building more energy than you're using.

So in the simplest terms possible, recovery from M.E. requires being primarily in a state of healing, but if we're dealing with this mysterious illness and no one can explain it, and you know you've got to pay the bills and you've got a family to support and all those stresses and anxieties, it can cause people to go into what we refer to as a Maladaptive Stress Response. So, their ability to handle and tolerate stress is now nothing like it would be in a normal person.

I: But, what is a healing state in practical terms? How does one live in a healing state?

A: It sounds like a simple question but there's a lot to it. I think the first thing is there needs to be a place of acceptance, and there needs to be enough support in the environment that someone is able to properly rest.

I: So, if somebody has a job and children to look after and the general things one has in life, then what you're saying is almost a question of discipline, saying I have to take time in the day just to be quiet. Is that what we're talking about?

A: Yes and it obviously depends upon how severely ill somebody is. So, if someone's in a category where they can just about keep going with their life, it may be enough to take time each afternoon for example to rest. If someone is very severely affected it may be a lot more drastic than that. Certainly we've found that if people can create a supportive environment and come to a place of acceptance, and start to treat the underlying physical things that are going on, that certainly creates a much more supportive environment.

I: So, I'm just wondering what practical steps people can take on board from what you've said so far. Let's say the average businessman, a person at school or a very active housewife, what should they actually do in terms of assessing their situation to see if they can make improvements?

A: I think that's a really good question. The first thing to say is that if there is more tiredness than should be there, there will be reasons. Often what happens is people will just go, "Oh well, I'm just tired..."

I: And you're saying that's not a natural state?

A: Absolutely not. If someone thinks that tiredness is not being able to do a 100 hour week then we've got something in their expectations to be looked at. But if someone's doing a reasonably normal day to day life, and they're feeling more tired than they should do, there will be reasons. As you mentioned earlier, it's a very obvious thing, but it also makes a big difference to actually listen to the body. So if somebody is at a certain time of day always feeling more tired, rather than just pushing through that, to actually listen to that. And, they may even notice that they feel more tired after eating a certain food for example. It could be a very simple thing that's going on.

I: So food can trigger an intolerance?

A: Yes, sure. Back in the 90's it was for a while seen as potentially the answer to M.E., but in reality I think it's only a small part of what is going on for most people. But, it could be that someone's built up intolerance to a food, and when they eat the food their immune system thinks that something's invading them and therefore they have a reaction to it. I am a great believer in people taking proper rest; you know proper rest doesn't normally mean coming home from work and crashing on the sofa and watching loads of mindless TV. It keeps the mind very active doing that.

I: And drinking beer or...

A: Yes. For anybody that doesn't believe that what we put in our mouth affects how we feel then I encourage them to try eating a load of chocolate for the day and another day eat something very healthy. There is a difference, and I think that nutrition has got a bit of a bad reputation because of people's resistance to the idea of changing their habits and how they live.

So really simple things that most people already know, like eating more vegetables, for some people will make a difference. This isn't obviously a curative treatment for M.E., but in terms of managing life: decent rest, eating basically healthy food (without necessarily becoming obsessive about it), and listening to our body, are all a good foundation.

I: So the starting point really is someone almost looking in the mirror and saying, "Look this is not really working, I'm heading maybe to a dangerous place, I've got to take stock, I've got to see if I can stop using too much of my resources and try to find more of a balance in life," and they have to try and make some adjustments if they can.

A: If you look at M.E., we can base what we do on one of two things: we can base it upon what our mind and the environment tells us, or we can base it upon what our body tells us. Now, in day to day life of course we have responsibilities and things that we have to do, but if we spend nearly all of our life being dictated to by our mind's conditioning and our environment, and we never listen to our body, after a while our body is going to start to shout, and if we ignore the shout it's going to start to scream. If we ignore the scream, then it's going to do something a lot more extreme which is often when chronic fatigue and M.E. occurs.

I: But you see our life doesn't support us with that. The other day I was getting some petrol for the car, and I fancied a little snack and I went down the various rows of food, and they're all basically unhealthy choices, packed full of sugar which would give me a temporary lift, that's true, but wouldn't actually solve the problem long-term. There wasn't one thing that I regarded as something healthy to eat, and so you really have to go against the grain.

A: That's true. I remember when I was a teenager I'd only eat two vegetables, which were peas and potatoes! I would sit there if I had to for three or four hours refusing to eat something that my family would suggest might be better for me. That only changed when after six months of struggling to get out of bed, I was desperate to try anything.

Coming back to what we were saying about when people become ill and we have these perpetuating factors such as the maladaptive stress response. It relates to what we were saying about when we're stressed all the time in our environment, and then you have something to really be stressed about which is an illness like chronic fatigue or M.E., after a while, the system starts to over respond to things. We talked about food intolerances and that's quite a good example.

If you think pre-September 11th, or before the London bombings, somebody could leave their bag on the underground and people would notice it and it wouldn't particularly be a big drama. People knew you were supposed to report a bag lying around prior to those events, but of course after those events people would have a much higher level of reaction to these things. I remember being on the tube soon after the London bombings and someone left a bag, and everyone just freaked out.

Now, this is kind of what's happening in the immune system for example with food intolerances that the body starts to react to things that aren't actually dangerous because it is in a heightened state of alert. And at the real extreme with chronic fatigue and M.E., we see this with light and sound intolerances, that people are actually living in darkened rooms with eye masks on because they just can't tolerate any light. The system's got so out of balance that it's reacting to things that just aren't dangerous. Also people that are watching this may start to notice that all these subtypes, trigger events, perpetuating factors and so on make this sound rather complex...

I: It sounds it to me!

A: Well, as we mentioned at the start, people are very used to having a specific pill for a specific ill and then to get better. And with all these different things that are going on, it's like being a detective, and people have to take that approach. But there are answers and there are biochemical reasons why people have their symptoms and, without going into too much biochemistry, there's the production of energy on a cellular level, and if the body's not reproducing energy efficiently, of course we're going to start feeling fatigue.

And this also explains to people who are watching this that do have M.E. quite a difficult symptom to understand, which is the delayed fatigue reaction people experience. For example, somebody can be doing a certain thing and they're aware they are pushing it, but they're kind of okay, and then it hits them two days afterwards, and suddenly it's like somebody has taken the plug out of them and the energy just disappears. This is because the body is not recycling ATP efficiently (ATP being the raw ingredient of energy), and when they crash it then takes a while for the body to then rebuild that cycle. And what this shows us is there are physical explanations of the symptoms that are going on. The trouble is it's different things for different people and that's what makes it so complex.

I: Yes, and as you were saying earlier, there's also psychological input that's causing those physical reasons as well.

A: Yes, so to try and simplify this information we've been talking about: you've got the predisposing factors, so you've got the things that are going on prior to developing M.E., and if you just had those, you may well never develop M.E. or chronic fatigue anyway. What you might have though is a bit more fatigue than most people. It might be that someone is always placing other people's needs first, like with the Helper subtype, and if they do that long enough, then after a while their body's energy is getting more and more diminished, and at that point if their way of being in the world is to help others, often they'll start to help others more because that's what they're used to doing.

209

I: So what a Helper needs to do is not only help other people, but also to help themselves sometimes.

A: Yes, but that's a very difficult thing for someone to learn to accept if they define themselves in that way. So we've got these predisposing factors, and then, for a percentage of people there's some kind of trigger event that happens, and we talked about things like a vaccination or a big event in their life and that causes the system to crash. But then you've got these perpetuating factors that we've also been talking about, and one of these being this maladaptive stress response.

We've got this whole new stress and anxiety of being ill and struggling to get through the day, and trying to explain to people what's happening, and thinking there's all these different ideas of what they should be doing. "Should I be resting? Should I be pushing myself through it? I'm on this special diet and I can't get the food," and so on. All this stuff just goes around and around in our head.

It's like the system has crashed, and when it crashes there is just nothing left to reboot it. It requires energy to heal, so if we're stuck in this stress state, there are no resources to start to heal and repair the damage of what's been going on.

I: I was also interested in how you dealt with this in your situation? I know some of it's in your book, but how did you deal with all this?

A: Initially not very well! But after several years of just being completely lost, completely overwhelmed and struggling to keep going with my life, I realised that if things were going to change, then I would have to do something to change them. I spent five years for myself consistently, and at times obsessively, researching health, psychology, nutrition, meditation - anything that I thought could make a difference.

I: So you had to build up your own picture of where you were and how you were going to change it by doing a lot of research. But you were motivated because you desperately wanted to get well. And that sometimes is the starting point. We don't want to be desperate. But when we are desperate, we're more willing to do something about the situation.

A: There's a huge amount of power that comes from desperation. And that's not just in M.E., we see it in all areas of life. But, in hindsight I was quite black and white about things, and maybe that was part of the problem. It was like my life wasn't worth living until I was well. Now, I'm not sure that was a particularly helpful way to look at it in some ways because it meant that I was always stressed any time I got a symptom, but it certainly drove a constant need to find answers.

Things that took me years to shift in those days, can of course now change a lot more easily with the huge advances in treatments both in the clinic that I run, and also with a few other clinics around the world that are doing ground breaking work. I spent five years studying and researching, seeing thirty-five to forty different practitioners from all kinds of different areas and I think at one point I was taking seventy supplements a day! I was doing all kinds of things like meditation and yoga to help with calming my system and so on.

I: So it was trial and error to a large degree?

A: Absolutely.

I: And what you're saying now is there is a lot more practical information and analysis people can find?

A: Yes. What I see happening is lots of practitioners, clinics and experts seeing so many more people with M.E. and chronic fatigue these days that it's driving people to research and understand it more. What we do very well as a clinic is look at what other clinics all over the world are doing and pull it together in an integrative way which takes the best of different treatments. And as I said before, there are reasons why people are ill, and there are treatments that work to get people better, but even now I'd be lying if I said to you that there's a magic answer that people come in and we do this one thing and everyone magically gets better. There are some patients that are still challenging to work with, but certainly for us as a clinic, they're the ones we learn the most from, and that's often where new discoveries and new ideas come from - when you've got somebody where you've done the things which generally would make a difference and they haven't. And that's from a scientific approach what through history has driven new discoveries, and it's a lot like being a detective: discovering what is really going on.

I: Is there ever a hopeless case?

A: It happens less and less, but there are cases of people we've treated for two to three years and they are only making what we consider fairly slow progress. But, we always hang in there with them, and we get there in the end. The interesting thing is that most people that come to us have tried a lot of different treatments before that haven't worked, so most people come in thinking they're going to be the hopeless case, and that's actually not true for the vast majority of people.

I: I think what I'm getting more and more from this is that people want to go to someone and for that someone to provide the answer. But, everyone is of course different.

A: And to be frank about it, it's not helped by practitioners, because the reality is practitioners' livelihoods are dependent upon having patients and treating them, and you know, if you go to a butcher and you say what shall I have for dinner tonight, they're going to sell you meat. If you go to a vegetarian cafe, they're going to sell you vegetables. Practitioners generally see the world through their model of how they see it, and therefore if you go to a certain practitioner for a certain therapy, they'll see it through their model, and they'll gather lots of information that their model's the model because that's how they're seeing it.

What we try to do is look at all the different models and try and pull the best together, and The Optimum Health Clinic's been going five years, it's treated thousands of people in over twenty-five countries, but we are using a new paradigm of treatment, pulling together different treatments, and it's a big project to understand.

I: So, what's the starting point? Someone has to make a decision, are they going to have to try and sort this out on their own? If you try and sort it out on your own, that's a tall order, but it's maybe possible - you did it! Or, people have to find someone near where they live, or someone that they can work with who can try and treat their case as an individual case, a special case, and see if they can find a way through this information.

A: Yes. It's interesting. I actually think it's both. There needs to be personal responsibility that's there, so when we treat people it's not that they give all the responsibility to us and it's our job to fix it. I think people always have to be their own practitioner to a point, but what they also want to do, is to work with people who are experts, not just a local nutritionist who's seen two or three patients with M.E. in their lifetime. We currently treat on average about sixty people a week with M.E. - there's a lot of knowledge that comes from that. One of the major benefits of the internet is that we have patients all over the world, because we can work with them using local laboratories where they are, and by doing things by telephone.

There's a heck of a lot more information available now than there was before. And I think it's really important that people understand that M.E. can feel incredibly isolating, and it can feel like it's never going to be possible to get better or to change it, and there are many, many people that have had M.E. and got better. It's different for everyone and it requires people to find their own path through it, but there are many inspirational stories of people who have had M.E. and got better, and it's really helpful for people to have access to those kinds of stories.

As you know, our philosophy as a clinic is to provide enough information for a person that is freely available to them to find out if it's going to be a fruitful way of them working on their own situation. This information is really key to peoples' understanding.

I: So if you were to just summarise, what are the main precursors for getting M.E., chronic fatigue and what are the main causes?

A: From our model, it is effectively a process of burnout. So, anything which causes the system to not be able to handle the demands placed upon it is a factor in causing M.E. It can be psychological traits (such as the helper, anxiety, achiever and trauma subtypes as mentioned), it can be physical traits (such as the detox, immune and structural subtypes), it can be environmental things (such as family, financial factors or toxic poisoning), it can be lifestyle things (such as poor nutrition) or it can be any combination of these factors.

In fact, just briefly, a very useful analogy is to think about a boat with different loads on it, and when you get to the point you have too many loads for the boat to be able to handle it and it starts to sink, that's really what's often going on with M.E. and chronic fatigue. Then you have a whole new load on this boat, which is the stress of being ill, so that's a useful way of looking at it, it's just too many things that are going on together.

I: And the way society is going, the boat's going to get more and more loaded up isn't it?

A: Yes. Well without getting too political here, one way of looking at it is the economy and the environment are getting their version of M.E. They've been out of balance for so long that the demands placed upon them are not sustainable. There has to be a readjustment, and that's one way of also looking at M.E. - it's a readjustment period that if used in the right way can actually be life changing in a very positive way, where people actually make changes that make their life a lot richer. It doesn't feel like that at the time I know, but it absolutely can be that way.

I: But isn't the planet getting M.E. as well? And this is not a joke!

A: Absolutely.

I: There are finite resources and they are starting to run out.
And even the banking system's got M.E...

A: Absolutely, absolutely. And you said it yourself earlier, the question is how quickly do we listen to that?

I: So it's really very much a question of listening to the messages outside, listening to the messages inside, putting it all together and living a life that is sustainable.

A: Right. That is not always easy when there are all these different demands on us. But, if we're able to find a way to do that, then ultimately life recovered from M.E. is often a much happier life than life prior to M.E.

I: So you see the M.E. situation that you were in that was very difficult at the time, as a positive experience now? So tell us more about that.

A: Yes, so I've gone on since my recovery to develop the clinic and that's been personally incredibly rewarding, to be able to help other people in a similar situation. But also in terms of a certain amount of self-insight and an ability to listen to myself and enjoy my own process through life. You know I didn't have a particularly easy childhood in

214

some ways, and I was conditioned to approach life in certain ways, and it's not really until we're forced to really look at that, that we actually make changes around that. And with people that we've treated at the clinic, it's often extraordinary the changes that come out on the other side that people discover after being ill, for sometimes decades. The things that seemed important before often don't seem so important afterwards, and often there are dreams or things people want to do in life that they never quite get around to doing, and M.E. really forces us to look at that. What do we really value in our lives?

I: It changes your perspective in a way?

A: Yes

I: Or, encourages you to change your perspective.

A: And, if people recover without making those deeper changes, often what can happen is there's a re-need for that wakeup call to take them back to living life in a more balanced way.

I: So they can recover and they can crash again in two years time?

A: If the underlying lessons and things aren't changed, sure.

I: It's a deep process isn't it?

A: Yes. I think we spend a lot of time in life wanting things to be different to how they are. We were doing a workshop recently for M.E. patients and people were saying, "I just want to get back to full time work," and I remember saying to them, "You know full time work is overrated sometimes!" I obviously don't miss having M.E., but there was something about having that time to really understand myself and to have that process and time can lead to some very important life lessons. You know we're always so focused on the destination of where we want to go and think we should be that if there's a place of finding happiness and joy on the journey to recovery, it's a very valuable lesson to have when we're recovered, because the challenges in life don't end when someone recovers from M.E...

I: No, I understand, it's ongoing. Ok, we have to wind up now Alex. I'd

215

just like to thank you very much for coming along. To remind our viewers that Alex and his team have a report that's available from his clinic called "M.E. in the 21st Century," and I like the subtitle 'You are no longer a mystery'.

That's a good point to end on. Thank you for watching Conscious TV, goodbye.

Nutrition and M.E./C.F.S./Fibromyalgia

Nutrition and M.E./C.F.S./Fibromyalgia
Alex Howard interviews Niki Gratrix (Director of Nutrition at The Optimum Health Clinic)

Alex: You're watching Conscious TV, and I'm Alex Howard. Today we're going to be talking about the role of nutrition in M.E., Chronic Fatigue, Fibromyalgia, and that whole group of illnesses. My guest in the studio today is Niki Gratrix, Director of Nutrition at The Optimum Health Clinic in London. Niki has treated over a thousand patients with M.E., Chronic Fatigue and Fibromyalgia, so has a huge amount of experience in the area. But before we come to M.E. specifically, Niki maybe you could start off by telling us a little bit about yourself, and how you got into working in this area?

Niki: Yes, sure. I'm a qualified Nutritional Therapist, but I didn't actually start out in this career. I had a prior life as a chartered accountant and was in banking and finance for about seven years, but I discovered during that career that it wasn't rewarding enough. I needed to have something that was much more heart connected and meaningful, so I cleared all of my debt, saved some money, and took a couple of years out. I got really interested in the whole mind-body connection, health, happiness, well being and basically the bigger questions in life. I did many, many different kinds of training all around the world, and then I finally said, right, nutrition's the thing I want to specialise in.

A: That's quite a big shift to have spent seven years in a career doing a certain thing and then to get to the point where you just decided that you wanted something completely different. It must have been quite a difficult decision and transition to make at the time?

N: It was and it wasn't. When I look back it definitely was. People would say that's very courageous to just have dropped a career after it took so long to qualify. But it's served me brilliantly, I use that material and the information that I learned in terms of running the clinic now. I didn't really know who I was when I was 21, 22, and by the end of my 20's, I'd found out who I was and what mattered, and what I really wanted to commit the rest of my life to doing, so it actually wasn't that difficult. M.E. is such a complex illness that actually you do need good logical and analytical skills to look at it, especially in the multi-factorial way we do as a clinic.

A: Along those lines, M.E. really seems to be an illness that has just confused doctors, psychiatrists, therapists and researchers with so many different opinions, from the idea that there's no answer, to the idea that there is some magic pill. Maybe you could explain a little bit from your experience, why it is that there's just so much complication around the area?

N: Well this illness has fallen below the radar of the orthodox medical approach. It challenges the orthodox paradigms of medicine. For example, I've got three things which I always talk about when I talk about M.E.; one is M.E. is a functional illness. What I mean by that is you don't just get ill one day out of nowhere. Health is on a continuum, and the continuum is between disease and optimum health, and M.E., falls slap bang in the middle of that. It's not a disease state that orthodox medicine would pick up on through any diagnostic testing, but it is far away from optimum health as well. So we call it functional medicine*, it falls right in the middle, that's where a lot of complementary and alternative practitioners work. It will keep getting missed by the medical profession, and it can make a huge difference when you treat that particular functional illness that falls in the middle. For example, we know a lot of M.E. patients are adrenally fatigued and the implication of that is that their cortisol will be too low, lower than optimum.

I've lost count of the number of patients that I'll treat where I've done some very sensitive testing on their cortisol level, found it to be suboptimal, treated it with nutritional therapy and the patient has amazing improvements. Quite a few of those patients would have gone to their GP, had a cortisol test done with an orthodox medical reference range, and the doctor every time will tell them that was normal and that there is nothing wrong with them, it's normal. The only time that an orthodox medical professional will probably tell you that there's a problem with the adrenals is if you've got Addison's Disease which is a diagnosable disease state. So that's the first thing that's really important.

A: And also when you talk about the adrenals, if you just explain just very briefly what their role is in the body.

N: Sure. The adrenals are an organ found just above the kidneys. Their main job is to produce the stress hormones, which are the get up and go hormones - the motivation and the energy hormones. When you've been very stressed for a long period of time, there are tonnes of those hormones pumped through the body. If that chronically continues for quite a period of time, eventually the adrenal glands will get fatigued and the level of the hormone production will drop through the floor.

So, it's these suboptimal states that are happening with M.E. and it's not only that. This is coming to the second principle in chronic fatigue. It's not just that one thing, or that one set of organs that are not 100% - it is multi-factorial. So it can be thyroid as well, there can be complications going on in the immune system, there can be low grade microbial infections, there can be metals' toxicity. All of these tend to fall below the radar and outside of the standard medical testing. It's a shame that people had all this going on when the doctors test them and they don't find anything wrong with chronic fatigue patients, and so they assumed for many years, "Well, OK, the patients must be making it up then - it's in their heads because all our medical tests show that everything's normal."

A: Which of course is very distressing to patients, to go in there seriously physically ill, and to be told there's nothing wrong with you.

N: It is terrible. Because, rather than saying, "Maybe we're doing the wrong tests and we need to change the tests we're doing," they were saying, "No it's nothing wrong with us, it must be the patients' fault and they are making it up." This has been the really bad news in the last thirty to forty years of the illness.

So you've got a multi-factorial approach and you've got suboptimal states. The orthodox approach doesn't really take a multi-factorial approach either. If you think about the standard medical approach it is very much that they look for one shot cures. They are interested in finding a single thing wrong in the body. Why? Because, it is usually treatable with a drug and it is the pharmaceutical companies that are mostly funding research and it is only interesting to them, when they find a one shot cure that they can promote as the pill that will cure M.E.

So you've got multiple system and organ imbalances happening, and there are actually clinics out there that have got this, but there is one last bit that they miss as well. They have got that it might be immunity, that it might be adrenal, that there might be mitochondrial involvement as well, BUT they forget that there's also the mind and emotions. So that's another system and impact in this whole picture. And at the clinic we look at suboptimal function, we use a multi-factorial approach, and we include the mind and emotions. Most medical doctors (even the ones who are saying they work holistically), really what they mean is they use different modalities on the body, but they are still not really working with the kind of techniques that we would use in the clinic.

A: I think also for many people affected by M.E., the idea of psychology playing a role is something very threatening to them given the years of misunderstanding from the medical profession. But, I know from your experience, working on the physical side, there is a very direct correlation between the mind and the body.

N: Yes. There are certain psychological techniques that are profoundly effective in treating chronic fatigue. CBT (Cognitive Behavioural Therapy) in our experience, those kinds of techniques are outdated. But, some of the brief psychotherapies that have come about in the last five to eight years have a profound impact on treating this illness. Not because it's all in the person's head, because M.E. is a mind/body event, because the two things are connected. What is going on emotionally and mentally impacts the physical body and vice-versa. We are not saying this is in your head in any way, shape or form. What we're saying is actually quite different. We are saying the two things are connected, and you can treat both.

There is definitely a chronic stress and trauma element that is at a higher level in M.E. patients than say somebody with M.S. and so on. For all of the reasons discussed, the medical profession hasn't picked it up. It would need a paradigm shift in their approach to how they approach health and disease, and that's why it's fallen below the radar.

A: Yes, and that's not just true of the medical system, it's also true of alternative practitioners as well - that people are looking for the one answer, and if we can treat this one bit then it's going to be a magic pill. What would you say about that?

N: When patients come and speak to us at the clinic in their free 15 minute chats (and actually I've probably done about three thousand 15 minute chats in the last four years), it's very informative because I've spoken to a huge array of different people with this illness, and you get to hear from them what's working, what doesn't work, and what their experience is of all the specialists out there. When people turn away from the medical orthodox approach because it hasn't been very helpful and they turn to the world of CAM (Complementary and Alternative Medicine), it's confusing. Do you do acupuncture, what about massage, and then you've got all these specialists in M.E. that are saying it's all one thing.

We have specific groups in the M.E. specialist world, like we have the microbe group, where it's a bacterial infection and you treat the bacterial infection and you can cure the illness, and then there's the individual practitioners saying it's actually just thyroid and adrenals, and you have other groups saying M.E. is Candida. So you've got all these specialists, and then you've also got all the other things out there like acupuncture and the rest of it which can be helpful, but aren't really curative.

Of course some people do benefit from working in each of these areas, but the problem arises when they tend to start saying, "This is what M.E. is, and this is THE answer". It gets messy and destructive again and confusing for patients because, if everybody is out there saying they have the answer, who do they believe? They could end up going through ten different practitioners to find out which thing worked for them because what's often happening is all these practitioners have a partial truth. They have a subgroup of M.E. people, and they are saying, "Yes it's all about adrenal and thyroid," another practitioner is saying, "It's all about a microbial infection and if you treat that, that's the key." Very often it is more than one of these things going on in a patient, and they need this multi-factorial approach.

A: And it also very much feeds into the standard idea that you have an illness, and you have 'THE cure' for an illness. That's also what patients, I think, often are looking for, and that's why they are so confused.

N: They kind of want a simplistic approach. It's very interesting. I went to the International Symposium on Functional Medicine this year that was taking place in California, and Dr. Cheney, who some people would have heard of as he has been treating M.E. for twenty-five years and is one of the leading clinicians treating this, had a very interesting story that he shared with the group. He had a patient, a very wealthy patient who was very frustrated with all of these problems in the M.E. world and who said, "OK, how can I get all you guys together, all you researchers, you specialists, all the people out there saying these different things, how can we get some kind of model together which is integrate?" So, Dr Cheney apparently said, here are all the leading experts in each of those areas, give them a first class plane ticket, fly them all into somewhere for a week together, chuck them in a room and see what they come up with.

So that is what happened; they got these experts from around the world, including Dr Cheney, people like Dr Rich Van Konynenburg and so on, and the most interesting thing that Dr Cheney said was that any time one of those specialists got up in front of the conference and said, "We have the answer to M.E.," the rest of the conference in his words "creamed them." There is a degree of megalomania that is bred of isolation, because there are a lot of researchers and practitioners out there that are seeing their groups, seeing lots of M.E patients, and maybe have one part of that partial truth, and are getting really amazing results with a subgroup of patients, but then not realising, that they've got quite a super select group that they're treating very well, but other clinics are using completely different treatments and might be getting the same level of results with a different group.

So it was great to hear that it is happening, that experts are stopping just saying that their way is the be all and end all, and are actually talking to each other and actually realising, "Oh this is multi-factorial - it can be more than one area." That's why there will be more work over time on developing subgroups, and that is what we are working on the at the clinic now: subgroups where we can say for example, "That person looks like they are high risk on say microbe and adrenal," so we immediately target treatment towards those, rather than just being hit and miss.

A: You know, it's interesting when you have different people that see it from their one perspective, and I think it's also linked into the fact that the business side of many clinics is built around them having a certain idea, and it's very difficult to have an open conversation with somebody whose financial security is dependent upon one way being THE way. Fortunately for us, our reputation is built on the integration of the most effective treatments available, rather than just one being the way.

N: There are many experts that have a lot to offer, it's just we all need to talk to each other more. It is moving in that direction, and the more of an integrated approach that we can get the better. I think some of these practitioners may be thinking they're getting better results than perhaps they are, and it reminds me of an article that was in CAM magazine about Candida....

A: And just to clarify Candida for those that are watching?

N: It's a yeast overgrowth in the digestive area and can become systematic and it can be a very important part in a subgroup of M.E. patients. But, there are some practitioners who are saying M.E. is Candida, and they expected their research results to have been better than they were. And, I think that's a common thing when we actually look at what results practitioners not working in an integrated way are really getting. They might be getting maybe 30-40% really significant improvement, but that's still only 30-40% and what's wrong with the other 60%? The key thing is you can work on one area and they might have three other areas that still need treatment, and they won't feel the difference until we've taken a multi-factorial approach.

A: Yes, but you know the interesting thing from what you're saying just at this point is such a contrast to what's out there in the standard medical system. You are actually saying that M.E. is treatable...

N: Yes.

A: You are actually saying that there are treatments that are effective (and there's obviously still a lot of clarification to be done in these areas and we'll talk specifically about some of these areas that seem to be effective), but you're saying that M.E. is a treatable illness?

N: It is.

A: ...and to some people that in itself is I think radical.

N: Yes, it's true. There needs to be more research, and we're definitely on board with doing that through the clinic's two year clinical trial we are about to start collecting data for. But, if you take one of the major studies already conducted in the area by Dr Teitelbaum (looking at

224

suboptimal imbalances and using a multi-factorial approach), although they have ignored the mind body thing, they were getting about 50% recovery rate and 46% significant improvement over a three month period.

A: In fact it's maybe worth saying at this point about where it's at in the UK in terms of research; I know you have looked a lot into the NICE guidelines where there is still so much of a focus on the psychiatric side.

N: I think because for so many years standard tests just showed there was nothing wrong, and so M.E. was a diagnosis of exclusion, which means there isn't a blood test or particular thing that you can get a positive or negative, and because nothing showed up, therefore by default you were diagnosed with chronic fatigue. So, because that's gone on for so many years and that was the history of it, that led to the conclusion it must be psychiatric. We need to identify subgroups and research those specifically. We need to replicate those studies. So, on the physical side there isn't enough evidence to justify the NICE guidelines being updated to include those yet. So all we are just left with is the psychiatric approach and CBT.

A: I know you mentioned to me recently a survey that was done of patients' feedback of what they said was helping them, and maybe it's worth commenting on that as well.

N: Yes, the M.E. charities are familiar with this. They've done studies of their own members, asking them what was helpful and what was unhelpful. One study that comes to mind is in 2001 one of the charities asked how helpful CBT was to members, and less than 10% said it was helpful, and with grade exercise 50% said they got worse doing it. They also looked at complementary therapies, including dietary changes, and 70% saw improvements.

A: And that's also just as a whole. People do all kinds of different things, nothing specifically targeted, but generally saying that this will benefit.

N: Exactly, and the conclusion being that that patients are saying these are helpful, but there needs to be well conducted studies to demonstrate this.

A: And, it's such a different paradigm of how to look at the whole thing. You've mentioned a few things, you've mentioned Candida and you've mentioned the adrenals; what are some of the other specific imbalances and specific areas that you find effective in treatment?

N: Yes. I'll mention a few and then we can go into detail with one or two that are most significant. The thyroid can be a significant area, but again it's how you are looking at the thyroid. We are looking for suboptimal imbalances, not so that the thyroid is so far gone that it's hit the reference range where the medical profession would diagnose low thyroid. We are talking about a low thyroid due to just nutritional deficiencies and things like Iodine and Selenium. There are also other parts of the endocrine system that we look at such as low growth hormones, some of the sex hormones as well, levels that are out of balance or suboptimal.

Digestion is a hugely important area, because step one is making sure people are absorbing the diet and the supplements and everything else we're recommending, so it becomes a hugely important area. The digestion's so hugely important because about 80% of the immune system cells are found in the gut. So if there are imbalances there, it's going to have an impact on the entire body. And you can't fix some chronic low grade bacterial or viral infections whilst the gut isn't sorted out. Another whole complicated part of this as well is intolerances and food allergies. We spend a lot of time looking into those areas where appropriate.

A: You mention the gut, maybe you could go into a little more detail around that and some of the symptoms that can be caused in that area?

N: Well everything in the body's connected. If you've got malabsorption happening - you've got pancreatic enzyme deficiencies, maybe low stomach acids and you are not breaking down your food properly - you won't be absorbing your vitamins and minerals properly. That can impact on every system in the body.

A: And I suppose someone could be eating the best organic food there is, but if there's no absorption of it then...

N: Yes, that's another reason why less experienced practitioners get confused. Step one for us is if we are going to recommend supplements is we need to first work on any gut issues to make sure patients can absorb them. That, and picking up infections, parasitic overgrowth, Candida and yeast overgrowth. C difficile is coming up a lot in patients at the moment, in fact that's reflecting some of the overuse of antibiotics in the last twenty to thirty years and what's going on in hospitals at the moment. So there are quite a lot of the bad microbes, and some of the parasites which can lead on to leaky gut (which is where the cells in the gut lining have got gaps that are too wide between them and that causes problems like food intolerances and so on).

So, there are some patients where pretty much the problems with their gut were the originating underlying predisposing factor which is how it led on to the illness developing into chronic fatigue. It is a hugely important area to understand as it links in with the immune system as well. We definitely know there are chronic low grade viral and bacterial infections that are systemic going on that go below the radar again. Those kinds of things can be actually key in some cases to making a difference. You can still sort out somebody's adrenals, sort out their thyroid, sort out their gut, but if you don't clear the low grade infections, the patient doesn't feel any different, so it's a really difficult process sometimes to keep patients on board with this...

A: What you're referring to, and maybe we'll come back to a bit later, is the different subgroups. There are some people from what you're saying that you could just treat the gut and that would be enough, and other people you treat the gut, and nothing would happen beyond that.

N: Yes. The other very interesting area that has had a big impact I would say in the last 4-5 years is also something called mitochondrial function. That has been a real key part of the picture to understand. It's not the be all and end all, it's not the final answer, and you can't break it down and say M.E. is mitochondrial malfunction, because there are reasons about why that went out in the first place and then there were secondary damages to things that happened because the mitochondria wasn't working 100%. But I'll just explain what that is and why that's an important part of the illness.

Your body has between 50-100 trillion cells. And practically every single one of these cells in the body has a little part in it, a little sub organelle called the mitochondria, and that bit of the cell is responsible for producing the energy of the cell, so that the cell can do its job, so it's got the energy to create proteins, to do its biological functioning.

I always use the analogy of a car engine: so it's constantly recycling, on and on, recycle, recycle. The thing that it produces is something called ATP, which is the energy currency of the human body, as it is throughout the animal kingdom. ATP is what the body uses to do the jobs it needs to do, and ATP is then sent back into the mitochondria where it is rejuvenated, where it is constantly recycled, so we literally have this circle of the recycling process. Now, if you think about chronic fatigue syndrome, you could pretty much say mitochondrial malfunction is probably the biological basis of poor stamina, so suddenly we have an understanding about when M.E. patients talk about experiences like "It felt like somebody just pulled the plug on me, I suddenly just had to go to bed and get sleep."

The other thing is delayed fatigue, where they will do an activity, and you might even be fine the next day or the day after, but then three days later, you are absolutely exhausted and wiped out and having to go and rest.

A: Which can be very confusing to the patient, because they've done that thing three days ago and they seem to be fine, and then suddenly their energy is just gone, seemingly out of nowhere.

N: Yes. So we can pretty much explain what is going on biologically in the body and we often spend time with patients explaining that to them, so they can understand what is actually happening on a cellular level. We have this recycling process going on in the mitochondria, and when the mitochondria are under-functioning, which can be due to toxicity, interference going on, a shortage of raw materials that the mitochondria need for energy production and so on, and what happens is the reserves and the speed of that production of ATP is under-functioning so a certain amount of activity will use up the reserves more quickly than in a purely healthy person. So suddenly the mitochondria have run out. I'm obviously simplifying this, but this is the experience of feeling like somebody has unplugged your energy system. You had low reserves, and if you put more demand on the physical body than the mitochondria is able to keep up with, that is the experience of somebody pulling the plug.

I don't want to get too technical because we could get really biochemical and that's not very useful in this context, but when you put too much demand on the mitochondria, ATP gets broken down to a different molecule, something called ADP, and then if you keep going and the demand on your body's going, going, going, that ADP is then broken down and lost to the body, the energy is literally lost to the body. That's why your body now has to create the raw materials from scratch, and that can take sometimes days, weeks, sometimes months to recover because ATP should be constantly recycled, ADP, ATP, ADP, ATP, but then if you put too much demand you can wipe your ADP out and then there are complications. The body is now making everything from scratch, and that's why it can take quite a while.

It's a bit technical but it really helps patients understand what's going on with that. It also helps them understand about why they may need the rest periods. From my experience, the power of the understanding of that with a patient is that they just calm down and they stop worrying about things so much, because they have learned what is going on in the body. They know that, for example when they've crashed, they know it is going to be fine, and they know that the body is just going to need some time to recycle and rebuild the energy reserves again. They can just do what their body needs them to do, and they don't worry and think this is going to be forever.

A: Yes. And it's also interesting that at the start you talked about M.E being multi-factorial, and there's an interesting correlation between the mitochondria and the adrenals, because you've got two different energy systems there: you've got your standard energy, and you've got your stress and your reserve energy. And maybe it's worth briefly explaining the relationship, because that shows how the different systems get affected, because if you're running out of your ATP energy, you're going to use your adrenals...

N: Yes, so when the mitochondria are down or are under-functioning, we do see patients start to live off their adrenal energy. Then they are living off nervous energy as well, and that can keep them going for a while, but then eventually the adrenals will probably go into an under-functioning state and crash as well, because all parts of the body need to work together. When there is an over stress of one area, different areas will crash and then we need to not just sort out the mitochondria, but then we've got the adrenals to sort out as well, so, yes, everything's interconnected and that's why it can be quite a complex thing.

For example, with the mitochondria, there is certain toxicity that can cause the problem, that can be linked to periods of stress that are allowing toxins to build up in the body. Then once the mitochondria are under-functioning, it's not just that direct explanation about the delayed fatigue and suddenly unplugging the system, there's a secondary damage that occurs from low functioning mitochondria, which compounds all the other symptoms. Mitochondria are actually found in huge amounts in the heart for example, so there's a lot of interesting research being done on the heart and M.E. patients as well. If your heart is sub-functioning, now you've got circulations not getting around the body, which leads to cold hands and feet and poor circulation. That is going to cause fatigue in itself, so each system that goes out can have a compounding effect on everything else, even though it wasn't the primary cause. M.E. is a process of things all interacting with each other in a feedback system, one affecting the other, so that's what I'm trying to explain - that it's not just a single one shop cure.

A: And, with the mitochondria being affected in that way, you talked about patients understanding what is happening so they can rest a bit more, but in terms of actual treatment, what are some of the things you can do to treat that?

N: There are for each different system and area, definite treatment plans, using dietary changes and usually different types of nutritional supplements. As a clinic we don't use drugs, and a lot of M.E. patients can have reactions to drugs and don't get on with them so we prefer a natural approach. We will be using certain vitamins and minerals supplementation, along with things like superfoods to make sure the basics are also right.

Macro-nutrition is basically fats, carbohydrates, protein, and then you have got your micro-nutrition such as vitamins and minerals. You've got to get all the basics in there right from the beginning, check that the patient is absorbing those things. Are they absorbing fats, proteins and carbohydrates? What is their vitamin and mineral status? And that is literally step one.

And, one of the things we do with every patient coming into the clinic is we get them to do ten or so tests they can get done with their G.P., which we know is nearly always going to come back normal from the G.P., and then we'll look at those test results using our own narrower reference ranges and we analyse them from a functional perspective.

A: What are some of those tests?

N: Things like liver function testing, electrolytes, thyroid testing, blood glucose, full blood count, all those kinds of things, and right from the start we can get an idea about just the basics. You know if someone is protein deficient and they are not absorbing protein properly, you can't rebuild and repair the body without basic protein. We said there are 50-100 trillion cells in the body, every single one of those cells has a fatty cell membrane, so if you're not absorbing your fats properly you will have issues with your cell membranes (the cell membranes control what goes in and out the cell).

So step one is, we just go right back to basics, and after that we go in for targeted organ support. That is the bit where we go "Right, do they need extra support for the thyroid and adrenals?" for example, and we'll work specifically using something like glandulars, which are actually animal extracts of that particular gland, that has shown to rejuvenate that gland and help it to get back up to optimal functioning. So that kind of targeted organ support. There are lots of different things we might do with the gut. We use a lot of probiotics, natural anti-microbial agents whether they are herbs or nutritional supplements.

A: We are talking about nutrition and M.E., and yet you're describing something so much more complex than that.

N: Yes. People often comment that the nutrition department is about a lot more than just nutrition. Dietary recommendations are fundamental to everything we do, as you need to get the diet right as it's the foundation that everything else is built on top of. One of the things we deal with on the diet side is if someone's got chronic allergies and food intolerances going on, then we get very specific about the diet and we look at if there are certain foods you need to avoid or rotate and so on.

But in terms of just the general guidelines on diet - we look at things like getting adequate protein in the diet, cutting the sugar out of the diet, the normal junk food stuff and the white refined carbohydrates. Often there can be a fundamental blood sugar imbalance going on that needs to be dealt with through diet, along with working on the adrenals, thyroid, immune system, and so on. We tend to fix that and get it sorted by step one.

A: And it's interesting you talk about getting adequate protein; I think a lot of people become a vegetarian with M.E. because they think that it's healthier for the system. What are your views on that?

N: People can recover from chronic fatigue if they are vegetarian, but being vegetarian isn't suited to all people. Basically it's coming back to the principle of biochemical individuality. There just isn't one diet that suits everybody. We do get patients sometimes who come in who are vegetarian and we can tell from their blood, the tests that we do and their symptoms of blood sugar imbalances (things like being starving hungry all the time, needing to eat every five minutes, being hungry even thirty minutes or an hour after a meal), there isn't enough protein in the diet for that person. The same amount of protein might work perfectly well for someone else, but isn't working for them, so we look at it very individually, there's no prescribed, "This is the diet for M.E. patients," - that doesn't exist.

Eighty percent of the time patients need to increase their protein intake based on looking at their protein levels in the testing that we're doing, and their symptoms. And protein is important for many things. M.E. patients need to be able to detoxify properly for they tend to have a back up of toxins in the system, because all the cells are going more slowly because of the mitochondria and so on. So when toxins are released, they often attach to protein to help them be taken out of the body, so protein is very important for that reason.

If we're constantly eating high sugar meals at points in the day, it causes large amounts of insulin to be produced, and insulin is the hormone that takes the sugar out of the blood and controls it and brings it back down. High insulin going on all the time can interfere with the detoxification. Also, the patient experiences this rollercoaster of energy levels during the day so they might feel great for about an hour after eating and then their energies drop through the floor, and then they need to eat again and they go up again. So there is this pattern of going up and down, that is usually related with blood sugar imbalances. What we tend to get sorted out earlier on is that we want at least the energy to be balanced. It may still be low because we haven't yet treated the adrenals and the mitochondria, but we tend to get that balanced out and that's important. For a lot of patients, carbohydrates and high sugar foods are not a sustainable energy source, they burn that stuff up really quickly. It's a bit like throwing hay at a fire, you get a fast explosion of energy, but it's gone very quickly. You want a slow burning log which is generally due to the proteins that sustain for longer.

A: This also leads back to what you were saying right at the start that there isn't any one answer or any one treatment, and not any one diet. Everyone is biochemically individual. But, it's interesting that the idea of the role of genetics in M.E. is something that's come up a little bit more over recent years, what are your thoughts around that?

N: There is some interesting research going on showing the C.F.S. gene or genes, so, you know they can be identified, which is important in the sense that if they do find certain genes in people diagnosed with C.F.S., it adds to the case that this is not just a psychiatric illness, but a genuine physical illness. But in terms of treatment for patients, I think we can get carried away, because at the end of the day even if they identify, "You have the C.F.S. gene," what does that actually mean?

A: I suppose what you're referring to is it is about gene expression. Someone can have the gene for something and not express it anyway.

N: Yes. So that's the thing, you are not predestined to get chronic fatigue just because you've got the genes. You have to have the predisposing factors which make that gene express, to then come down with the illness. So ultimately, the patient is still in control here, because they ultimately control the environment. If you create a toxic, stressful life and are in an undernourished and under-loved environment in your body, it changes the environment in the cells which allows those negative genes to express.

As we've already said, the orthodox approach tends to try and look for one shot cure, a single drug that would switch off the problem. If you think about what we've talked about, about all these factors that affect it - the multi-factorial impact, and the fact that it's a process of the interaction between the environment and all these different systems, mind and body - the idea that one gene could be switched off and that would cure the illness is just overly simplistic.

Also, if we get a little bit spiritual here, M.E. can be an experience, an opportunity. It's a wake-up call. Have I been living my life in the way I want to? How about my environment, both from a pollution point of view, as well as family, job and everything else? It is a wake-up call to look into all of those things, and if you just went to the doctor and said, "Can you give me a pill for this please," and then all that's gone, it takes away the opportunity for healing and actually having a transformative experience. And, many patients come out of their experience with M.E. and say it was the best thing that ever happened to them. Some patients will definitely find that extraordinary at the moment, but it is possible that patients can say that.

A: It's interesting because you talked at the start about your career change, your journey from working in corporate banking into the work that you do now, and what drove that change was the dissatisfaction inside of yourself and what you're really referring to with something like M.E., often it is a drive for someone to really explore themselves in these ways. So for people that are watching this and thinking, "Well, that sounds interesting, but it also sounds really complex," what are the next steps for people to find out more about this and for people watching, is there anything they can do at home? Where can they go with this?

N: There is a lot of free information on our clinic website. We welcome patients to go on there, and read in detail about specifics on how we treat the illness and how we approach it on both sides of the clinic, which are the psychology division and the nutrition division. There are also great patient recovery stories, interviews on specific aspects of the illness, tonnes of information on there. So, go and have a look at that to begin with, familiarise yourself with it. There are lots of things to discover on there. There's also an opportunity to sign in and get a free 15 minute chat with one of the practitioners in the clinic.

A: OK, we've got a couple of minutes left, what do you think about people who are thinking this all sounds great, do I just go and see a local nutritionist or find a book that recommends supplements, do you support people doing self-prescription?

N: It's really tricky because, to anybody who's out there, and I say this a lot in my free 15 minute chats as well: if you're going to see a practitioner in the alternative area for treating chronic fatigue, I would always recommend, go to see somebody who is at least specialising in the area. There is a huge difference between speaking to a practitioner who maybe treats one or two M.E. patients a year, to somebody who is doing this full-time. It's not comparable to the level of understanding for somebody who specialises in it.

A: In the final bit of time we've got left, what do you hope the future holds for M.E. as an illness, where do you see it going over the coming years? It's obviously accelerated hugely over the last five years even.

N: Yes, I think chronic fatigue is a challenge to the medical profession because I think it's between 0.2 and 0.4% of the population have chronic fatigue but I've seen research that suggests it's more like 1.5-2.5 million people just in the UK. 80% goes undiagnosed, so there could be another 80% on top that have got the illness, and I think this illness is on the increase. It has to be a wake-up call to the medical profession. If they want to fix this illness they've got to start from a different paradigm of understanding about health and disease, and I hope that that's what this illness will do. It might help to wake-up the medical profession to start thinking a bit more about the bigger picture.

A: To be less reductionistic I guess.

N: Less reductionistic, more understanding about a biological systems process rather than these simplistic one shot cures funded by pharmaceutical companies. So I also hope that the complementary and alternative medical approaches will get more validity. We, as a clinic are trying to help that. My aim is that we'll prove that what we're doing is working scientifically, and to show that the answer doesn't always have to be a drug, that other things aside from drug therapy have a hugely powerful impact for health.

A: Brilliant. Well thank you Niki for your time, and thank you for watching Conscious TV and hopefully we'll speak with you again very soon.

* Please note where Niki refers to ME/CFS as a "functional" illness she is using the word in the U.S. context as it is used by the Institute for Functional Medicine (IFM) who state that many chronic diseases involve imbalances in fundamental underlying physiological processes or biochemical "functionality". There are many imbalances

of functionality found in CFS/ME patients, and in some there have been serious physiological abnormalities found. Please note she is not using the word in the context it is used in orthodox medical circles in the UK where "functional" tends to mean a psychosomatic or non-biomedical kind of illness.

Psychology and M.E./C.F.S./Fibromyalgia

Psychology and M.E./C.F.S./Fibromyalgia
Alex Howard interviews Anna Duschinsky (Director of Psychology at The Optimum Health Clinic)

Alex: You're watching Conscious TV, and I'm Alex Howard. My guest in the studio today is Anna Duschinsky, Director of Psychology at The Optimum Health Clinic in London, and today we are going to be talking about the role of psychology in M.E., Chronic Fatigue, Fibromyalgia and that whole group of illnesses.

Anna, before we come to psychology and that area, maybe you can start off by telling us a little bit about your background and how you came to work in this area.

Anna: Yes, sure. I guess the quick answer is I work in the area primarily because I myself had Chronic Fatigue or M.E., some years ago now. I was about thirteen when I got glandular fever from a boyfriend who had it for about two weeks; I never quite forgave him when I had it for about ten years! And from that point onwards I just kept getting ill. I had tonsillitis very regularly, and remember being in and out of the doctors, but no-one was really mentioning C.F.S. or M.E. at that point.

A: So you were going to school, struggling to keep up and going down with colds, flu and that kind of thing?

An: Exactly that, I was regularly missing bits of school - I remember escaping home in free periods - and that had been entirely out of character for me up until that point. I was also missing a lot of social time. I became notorious for not going to any of the parties that I was invited to, which was not a reputation I wanted! I was just finding it really tough, particularly as it got towards GCSE's and then A-Levels. We really had no idea what was happening, and I kept going to the doctors and just being told, "It's glandular fever again and it's just a recurrence of the same thing."

A: It must have been incredibly challenging. At that age especially, when you are used to going to the doctor, getting a pill, and getting better. What was the point where things on your own healing journey started to turn around?

An: Well, they get a lot worse before they got better for me. I made it to university, but very quickly began to get a lot worse. I decided I was unfit, so took up rowing, which really was not the best idea, getting up at 5am in the morning and going rowing, so quite quickly I crashed very severely, and spent about a year in bed.

That was the year I decided there was definitely something going on and I needed to look at that. The doctors were just offering antidepressants, and essentially telling me to go home and sleep. At age nineteen I decided that should not be my life, and I started to take it into my own hands. I started to read around the subject, reading a lot around nutrition, health, and psychology, and I started to piece together the jigsaw-puzzle of what it was that was really going on for me.

I guess that was the point, after that really bad year, that I started to turn things around. It took a little time for me to get to the point where I'd fully recovered, because I was pretty much making it up as I went along, and attempting to finish a degree in the process. So that was a big part of the motivation to continue to work in this area - that it doesn't have to be that difficult, because at times it was such a challenge for me.

A: Obviously we'll talk about psychology in the interview today, but it must have been quite a difficult thing at that point to embrace the idea that your psychology and your thoughts were causing this very physical situation you were in? How did you come around to that idea yourself?

An: It's a good question and I really relate to my patients now when a part of them wants to hit someone when they talk about the psychology side, because the connotation of psychology for many people is that it means they are just making it up, and that is really tough when you've been through years often of feeling really physically ill, you can't walk to the supermarket, you can't do all the normal things in life. There is no question that something really physical is going on.

I think it was just reading a lot around the subject, and beginning to understand that the concept of a Cartesian break between head and body (that mind are body are completely separate), just isn't accurate. And, realising that the way you are thinking and feeling emotionally massively impacts on the way you feel physically as well. So that, bit by bit, began to leak into my consciousness, so I started to think differently and feel differently about it.

A: So with the transition of your own journey, and then coming to work with others, talk to us a little bit about that transition and getting more and more interested in this field and the different tools, because psychology is a big term, and there are lots of things that are part of that.

An: Sure. I guess, I'd never considered being involved in this area prior to that at all. I was doing French and Italian at University when I got ill.

A: Rather a different direction.

An: Slightly different! Still about communication as you look back on it, but not the same at all, and I think it really was the recognition of how much it had helped me, and then realising that I'd been fairly lost up until that point in terms of what I really wanted - I was just kind of on the treadmill. I did my GCSEs and did pretty well, and did my A-Levels, and went to University, without really any idea of where I was going in my life. And M.E. in a way is a gift (easy to say in hindsight I know), where you can step back and review your life and who you are.

So, I realised that what was really interesting to me was psychology and how people worked, and how the mind and body impacted on each other. The tools I chose to train in are very much the sort of brief therapy end of things, so very much the practical and solution-focused way of looking at psychology and behaviour, and that's because that is what made the biggest impact on me. So, things like NLP (Neuro-Linguistic Programming) which we'll go on to talk about in a bit, and those kinds of tools, seem to me, to make the most difference. It was a really interesting transition. I trained in all of this because I was fascinated, and I had an idea it would be good to work with people who had been ill, but really had no idea if I could, until some friends of friends started to come out of the woodwork, telling me that they were ill with M.E. and saying, "Well you've recovered, and you've trained in this stuff, can you help?!" And I said, "I have no idea." So, I spent some time working really pro bono with increasing numbers of people and kind of got to the end of six to nine months, reviewed and went, "Ooh, they're getting better; there must be something in this." So, that is the point I really began to think about this seriously as something I could work with.

Psychology M.E., C.F.S. and Fibromyalgia

A: You mentioned that on the psychology side it doesn't mean that someone is just making it up and maybe it's worth talking a bit about the difference between the conscious and the unconscious, and how just because there is a mind-body component, it doesn't mean that they are crazy or that they are making it up.

An: As we'll go on to talk about, the connection between the mind and the body are very real, physical factors. If you're in stress, the way that impacts your physical body is extraordinarily real and chemical. It makes significant chemical changes to what's going on in your body. So, whereas we might say that we're making it up or it's all in the mind, there are entire branches of science now looking into this as a concept, and proving that mind versus body really is a very outdated way of thinking. What we really need to look at is how our psychology can impact and control what is happening in our physical body, and that's just a massive factor in this kind of illness.

A: And that's also quite different I think to how a lot of people may be seeing it, there's been talk about a lot of genetics and that kind of thing. What are your thoughts around that?

An: If we're talking about illnesses like Chronic Fatigue, we know that there's got to be a genetic component, without a doubt, because otherwise, why did you get M.E. as opposed to something else? And in fact, we all know people who really should have burnt out by this point given the way that they are pushing themselves, but they haven't, so there must be genetic components underlying why we choose physiologically to express this through M.E. rather than through something else.

But even in illnesses like breast cancer (which we know to be significantly genetic), I think the statistics I read recently is that it is around five percent due to genetics, which is very, very low if you think about it, and lower than most people would expect. I think the key thing to realise is, yes, there's a genetic component, but genetics don't dictate what happens. It is the genetics plus all of the lifestyle factors and triggers that go on top of that which dictate whether or not you get M.E. or C.F.S. or you don't. So, it's a factor, but I don't think personally that it's the answer. It just gives us more information.

A: You're talking about the role of the mind and the body, maybe it's also worth explaining a little bit about how that actually interlinks. I know you do a lot of work with people with stress states and healing states, and maybe explain a little bit about how all that works, because I think a lot of people say things like "I was always stressed in my life before, but now I don't have to go to work any more because I've got M.E., how can I be stressed?"

An: Absolutely. We tend to think of stress as something that happens in stressful situations, and I guess the key thing to understand is that human beings are built for stress, very much; we are designed to work with stress. But we're designed to work with caveman stress!

A: Do you want to explain what you mean?

An: I will. If you think about being a caveman (because in essence we aren't that physiologically different to how we were in those times), cavemen will have wandered around in the bushes, picking berries, and at certain points in the day or the week they would have come up against a real physical threat, such as a big woolly mammoth or a sabre-toothed tiger. At that point, the system is triggered into stress, and the adrenals pump out adrenaline in the body, and your muscles work differently so you can fight, flight or freeze, and physiologically everything changes in the body for that time. That's absolutely OK if all you're doing is running away from a tiger or fighting it off: that's not going to take that long, so it's a fairly short-term state to be in. And what will then happen is the body will normalise again. It will adapt back to the fact that you're now just wandering around the bushes again.

So, we are designed to handle what's called acute short-term stress very well, and some people find they work best under those conditions. In fact, actors always say that if they don't get a little bit nervous, there is something wrong. What isn't so good for us are the ongoing stresses. Most of us don't live like cavemen any more; our stresses are ongoing day-to-day stresses that are there a lot of the time.

All of the patients I've ever seen with M.E. have had ongoing chronic stress in the period coming up to getting ill. The problem with that is that we weren't built for it and it's completely unsustainable for the body to maintain that fight or flight state on an ongoing basis, because your adrenals weren't designed to work that hard. Your entire body wasn't designed to be in that state. Things like the immune system are suppressed in that state, your digestion doesn't work well in that state, because they are not important if you're fighting a woolly mammoth, right?!

A: I guess digesting lunch is not a priority at that point!

An: No, so what we're saying is: if over a long period of time your body is subjected to that state, it will start to have a severe detrimental impact on your health. And we've known that since Hans Seyle in the 1920's did some experiments with rats under chronic stress. Not that we're advocating that in any way, but that was really the beginnings of our understanding the impact of stress on the body.

A: So what you're saying is that often in advance of M.E. there are too many stresses that are happening in someone's life together, and it's almost like the overload of that which then becomes the issue?

An: Exactly. It is the overload. And the problem with that is because the body's overloaded it thinks it still needs to be in stress. It determines that you're under threat, because physically and emotionally you are under threat from all of these stresses. And, the body learns to consider this state of stress as being normal. So exactly what you say, a lot of people come into clinic and they say, "Yeah, I was stressed when I first got ill, but since then I've done nothing for weeks, months, or even years, why haven't I got better?" This state is what we call the "maladaptive stress response" - which is, if you put someone in chronic stress over an ongoing period of time, the body learns to stay there. It doesn't adapt back to the healing state in a way that it should, and the problem with that is that you could be doing nothing, but be very stressed.

A: And also having an illness like M.E. is incredibly stressful. So people have got the stress of also being ill.

An: It's one of the most stressful things I would say. It's even more traumatic because as you said at the beginning when I was going through my experience, I was expecting doctors to say, "This is the way that you come out of this and this is the problem, and this is how long it will take, and take this pill and you'll be better," and that's the old model that we expect from the medical system. Of course M.E.

utterly doesn't fit that model, so there's a lot of stress around being ill in itself and what is happening. There are all these weird physical symptoms and often we are not able to explain it to friends, family, partners, colleagues and so on. It can often feel like you are living a double life, and that is incredibly stressful and quite traumatic for people that are going through it.

So, as you say, even if there were no stresses before it, having M.E. is incredibly stressful and the problem is of course in that state, your body is not acting in a way that is going to be helpful for actually healing and getting well. The clue is in the name: "Stress state and healing state." And actually, you've got to be more in a healing state more of the time for your body to get well, and the situation and the circumstances of M.E. often mean we're in stress most of the time.

A: Yes, it sounds like what you're saying is people are effectively in exactly the opposite state to what they need to be in to be able to heal. It's like the story of the frog: if you put a frog in a glass of cold water and heat it up it will stay there and die. But, if you drop it in boiling water it will jump straight out again and live. People have got so used to being stressed, they don't even realise how much they are in that state.

An: Absolutely, and I think the key thing to realise is our body knows how to be well. Our body knows how to heal. At least I very much believe that that's the case, and I think that if you aren't healing, and you've stopped and taken away the original stresses, then what we know must be the case is that at some level your body isn't in the right state to do it. It's still acting as if it's running away from tigers all of the time, and I think most people with C.F.S., M.E., Fibromyalgia recognise that to be true, because if they really stop and think and feel into their body that is often how it feels.

A: Yes, and I guess maybe it's also worth at this point explaining a bit about how this also relates to the physical side of it. I know you're not saying that it is just chronic stress that is going on, and maybe it's just worth talking a little bit about the interrelation of the psychology side with some of the physical factors that are going on.

An: It's kind of cyclical and it's a bit of a spiral. We've developed in the clinic a model integrating the nutrition and psychology departments to show how all of this really fits together. Just to go through that a little bit briefly. I guess you're starting with genetics as the underlying factor and on top of that we looked at some of what we call the subtypes.

What we mean by subtypes is really predisposing factors that make you more likely to get ill, and those can be both physical and mental or emotional. For example, psychological subtypes could include people who were always real worriers and anxiety types, or people that have always looked after everyone else's needs before themselves (the helper type), people who define themselves by their achievements, and those who have experienced trauma.

Equally there are physical subtypes. So, having a really poor diet and not really looking after yourself; in other words, diet and lifestyle factors. Or people who do shift work, which can really disturb the balance of the whole system. Also, some people will know that from really early on they had immune issues. They were always getting sick or they always had allergies, that kind of thing. So we know that underlying everything else, those predisposing factors will make you more likely to get ill. So, as I say those can be either physical or psychological, or both, and usually it's a bit of both.

You talked about overload, and we sometimes describe it as a bit like a load on a boat. The loads and triggers will tend to be both psychological and physical. And of course one predisposes you to the other, so the more your system is in chronic stress, the more things like the digestive system and immune system tend not to work as well - so you are making yourself susceptible on a whole range of levels. If I look at my own story, the other factor to what was happening at the time, was that I was thirteen to fourteen, pretty competitive and stressed and working hard, and had been very much into dance. So, unfortunately, like so many thirteen year old girls, I had stopped eating properly and was starving my body of the nutrients it needed. My point is that it was not ONE issue, but a whole set of factors going on the period of time that gradually led to the slide down into chronic fatigue.

A: It's a different era now isn't it? Thirteen to fourteen years old and being stressed having too much to do!

An: I know - crazy but true. And I think that all of these things interlink: so the chronic stress, plus some of the physical loads that start to happen, diet and all sorts of physical bugs and viruses, and not really absorbing things properly, and starting to get food allergies or intolerances - all of these things together, build the load on the boat, and that is really what "causes" M.E.

In my view, M.E. and C.F.S. are really burn-out; they don't have single pathogens - they are more of a gradual, developed "state." Some people can identify some significant triggers - but even then, we are looking at the 'final straw that breaks the camel's back' - there has almost always been a lot of background even prior to that point.

A: And also, so far, we've talked about the role of psychology and the mind, but it's also maybe worth talking a bit about the role of emotions, so what do you see as being the role of emotions within this whole picture?

An: I think that, for a lot of people in their day-to-day lives, they can be a little bit disconnected from their body and their emotions. Very often if we're focused on achieving and doing the best in our job, or being the best mum or being the best wife, or the best husband or whatever it is, we are very often focused outside of ourselves, and we're not giving a lot of time or attention to what's happening inside of ourselves. Now, if we are emotionally disconnected, we are not necessarily looking after our own emotional needs, we are not looking after our own physical needs, these two kind of go together - we are just not paying attention. And, in a way, that has to be the case for us to get ill.

I often think of it as being a bit of a relationship, so you have a relationship with your body, and very often by the time you've got to burn-out, that relationship is in tatters. You haven't been talking, you're not listening to each other, you hate each other, and you're not working well together - that's really the relationship we've often built up towards our self.

A: And I guess that for most people at that point the relationship gets even worse because it's now, "You're not supporting me, you're not there for me" and everything else.

An: Exactly, because you know, suddenly your body's not doing what you want it to do.

There has often been a fair amount of build up to getting ill emotionally in terms of events and triggers that have gone on. And, because we're so focused on trying to keep everything going and juggle all the balls and keep it all OK, we sometimes don't give ourselves time to even process what's been going on. Quite often people will have triggers of losing a loved one, or a relationship break up, or something happening in their life that does deeply impact on them emotionally, but maybe they are not really giving themselves the time and resources to deal with it. So those factors tend to mean that part of the process of healing is really a mental, physical, emotion and spiritual state of balance. You've got to get a level of balance with yourself again emotionally to create health again, so that's part of the process of healing I think.

A: I think for a lot of people it may be a new idea that not being in touch with their emotions can be a factor in this whole disease state that is going on, so maybe it's worth explaining a bit about some of the physiological ways that the mind and the emotions are impacting the body.

An: In really simple terms, I guess you can look at your body as being the seat of your emotions, and when we don't pay attention it can be a little bit like we cut everything off from the neck down. Your unconscious mind has a prime directive to keep you safe and keep you well. It also has a level of wisdom, and maybe that's a new idea to some people, but we're quite used to in our culture and language to thinking of the idea of a "gut feeling," we talk about that a lot, or being "heartbroken," we do actually have a sense I think in our culture that intrinsically our body does have an intelligence to it: that there is a deeper intelligence than just the mind. And one of the ideas that helped me a lot in getting well was that actually, my body wasn't just trying to piss me off by getting ill! It wasn't just a physiological machine that had gone wrong, but almost this process was trying to tell me something about what was happening in my life at that point, and who I was being and how I was being. Partly that was physically not taking care of myself, and the body's going to tell you that.

A: I think it's interesting what you say about the body having its own intelligence, because when you really think about it, it's extraordinary how complex the human body is, and yet people treat it like it's an ignorant thing which has just suddenly gone wrong and broken down.

An: We perceive our bodies to be machines. And you can blame the last couple of hundred years of science. They've done fantastic things for us in many ways, but it has turned into a mechanistic view of the body, which is why the medical system works in this way today. You know, you have immunologists who look at one part of the machine, and endocrinologists who look at another part of the machine, and actually it's a whole system. We increasingly understand that the mind and the body are the same system as well. You can emotionally experience something and your cells experience that too.

So it's beginning to look at your whole body as a very intelligent system. We still have no idea how quite a lot of the body works, even despite the amount of research that's been done. It's beginning to respect the body as more than a machine, and understand that at the point where we burnout, that isn't an accident. There has been a whole series of things happening; we've talked about the triggers and the facets and the factors that go into that, but also that the intelligence of your body is literally saying, "Hang on, stop, this is not getting you where you want to go" and, if you look at it, it's a bit of a wakeup call. It's a part of us asking us to pay attention, and it's a great analogy to imagine it a little bit like a phone ringing, designed to get your attention.

And, if you don't listen to what's emotionally and physically happening on a small scale, your body will keep intensifying your symptoms to get your attention. For most people with M.E. or C.F.S., if you really sit back and look, there were always indications, emotionally and physically that this was coming.

A: Yeah, and I think for a lot of people this can be very difficult to take on board, but hopefully with the way that you are explaining it, people will recognise that it also makes a huge amount of sense.

There are obviously a number of different psychology based treatments that are out there which have attempted to help with M.E. with, I guess limited amounts of success in some cases, but maybe it's worth talking about just a little bit about CBT (Cognitive Behavioural Therapy) which is the main traditional psychology treatment used?

An: CBT is a very useful tool for understanding the role of the mind in behaviour and the creation of behaviour. But, CBT has to my mind one key drawback, which is that it works primarily on a conscious level - it works to retrain the conscious thinking patterns, and we find in the

248

clinic that a good deal of what is happening is conditioned, unconscious triggered behaviour. In other words, working with the conscious mind is a start, but not enough.

The other key issue with CBT in the way that it is being used by the NHS - and of course, this is a generalisation, because different practitioners and services will be working in different ways - is that it takes a very reductionist view of what is happening. From what I see, this can actually operate in two very different ways - either the message that patients are getting is that M.E. is purely physical, and so the CBT is there to help them manage and deal with the response TO the illness, rather than with any expectation of actually helping that much in terms of physical recovery; OR the message that the patient is being given is that it is all in their minds, and there is nothing physically wrong except for their reaction to what is happening around them - and this too is over-simplified for what is in reality a complex illness.

A: And alongside CBT often goes graded exercise and pacing also. Maybe some of your thoughts around those treatments?

An: I think both really have their place, but the problem with M.E. is that it is an umbrella term for basically lots of subsets of what's going on. For some people, beginning to pace their activity, by which we mean do a certain amount of a certain activity followed by resting, followed by a certain amount of a different activity, followed by resting and really getting very, very formalised with that, can be helpful. It's usually helpful for people who had a tendency to completely ignore their body, and race ahead and do everything they could and pay no attention to themselves.

So in this case, for this subset of people it will make quite a lot of difference, but it very often won't get them the whole way. For others it can become a problem, and what I mean by that is we see a lot of people who have been put on very strict pacing regimes where the pacing regime takes over their life, and in fact because intrinsically we talk about part of the core issue as being stress and anxiety, if you have to pace really rigidly, and you're already stressed, it becomes another source of stress. The danger is also we want people to learn to listen to their bodies, and pacing effectively causes them to stay in their head. So pacing can be useful but is very limited.

A: So it's almost like it can break somebody out of boom and bust (overdoing it and then crashing), but you are also saying that if someone can only speak on the phone for three and three quarter minutes for example, which we've actually come across things as extreme as that, then if someone's on for even another ten seconds, they can then go into anxiety worrying that they're overdoing it and they are doing too much.

An: I have had patients who are timing to the second with stopwatches, and it became a massive feature of their anxiety that they feared they couldn't do more, and that very fear meant that if they went a few seconds over, their whole system would spring into high, high stress, which is not very helpful obviously when we're talking about being in a healing state as opposed to a stress state. So that's a facet of it. I think the other thing to say is we talked about body intelligence, and a lot of my learning was that my body had a sense of what was right for it in any moment. If you think back to far more simple times, then intrinsically, we are at some level animals; that's what we came from, and animals don't think about what to eat and when to eat, they just do it instinctively and naturally, and we instinctively and naturally know when to eat and when to stop, and when to rest and what we need and far more complex things than that. So, my sense of 'pacing' is that it is the process of learning to listen to those real, instinctive signals - and so as you say, although strict pacing regimes can initially help to break the cycle, it is not a long-term solution or the whole answer for most people.

A: How about graded exercise therapy (GET), which has had a huge amount of negative press from a lot of M.E. patients, and in many ways for good reason?

An: Again, I think you've talked a little about nutrition in other programmes and the different kind of physical things that are going on. For some patients, beginning to gradually build up exercise at a certain point in their recovery can be helpful. But, the problem is for a lot of people, the body is still burnt out and you are still in this stress state most of the time. Physically there can be all sorts of things like adrenal fatigue and mitochondria malfunction, and it's a bit like trying to push a car uphill without petrol. There are no resources there to use.

You've got to get the body into the right state before you have the energy to actually start to exercise. And for those who are still very burnt out, and still have significant issues going on in the physical body, then pushing further - exercising - is probably going to be counter- productive. And of course, if the body is still significantly in stress for the majority of the time, then exercise just adds another 'load' to the boat. The key really, is on an individual basis, to understand the different factors at play, the stage of the illness that you are at, and then from there to be able to judge what it is that you need at that point to heal. Exercise is one factor that will play a part, but only at the right time and given the right conditions.

A: So what you're referring to is different things at different stages of the illness. A treatment which has become quite well known over recent years, partly because of the first edition of my book "WHY ME?" is the Lightning Process. Again, this is something that works at certain stages for certain people, and maybe it's worth again just briefly talking about that.

An: Exactly that, and I think it's almost quite similar. For some people, I think from my experience it is quite valid to say that the stress and anxiety of being ill has become the major issue in itself. It is, as we have said, quite traumatic, and for some people who often have already a tendency towards anxiety, the symptoms, the limitations and uncertainty of M.E. engender such fear that this really takes over. We have talked about the maladaptive stress response, that state where the body gets 'locked into' the fight/flight/freeze state, and fails to normalise out of it. Well, in this condition, the body will not be functioning normally, and there is no question that for some people, fear of what is happening with the illness is the key factor in keeping that maladaptive stress response in place. If that is the primary issue - and for some it is - then The Lightning Process can be effective at breaking the fear patterns and enabling people to 'normalise' back to living their lives again. That is where you are seeing the 'miracle cures' - there is nothing especially miraculous, they have just dealt with the anxiety.

The trouble is for people who actually have anything else happening - and by that we mean the subsets where there are more severe physical imbalances, or even more engrained emotional issues which need to be looked at, they will be encouraged to use The Lightning Process to push through all of this - and we see people who either are made worse, or relapse later. If there is a good deal of physical imbalance, then pushing through is only going to work either short-term, or not at all. And if you have emotional patterns of pushing yourself, for example, then you will be effectively repeating the same pattern that got you ill in the first place; it doesn't address what's gone on emotionally and doesn't teach people to listen to themselves. So the Lightening Process sells itself as a solution for everyone with M.E. - the reality is far, far more complex than that.

A: So you're saying that some of the ideas and tools in there can be helpful but in a more integrated format of using it?

An: That would be my view, that in a way it is dealing with again one factor, one facet of M.E., without seeing the whole picture, and you really have to see the whole picture I think.

A: And another treatment approach which also had a lot of press a few years ago is something called Reverse Therapy (RT). Again, just explaining briefly what that is and some of your thoughts around it.

An: We've talked about the body and the intelligence of the body, and the idea that there is an emotional intelligence and a real fundamental wisdom there, and I think that is very true and it was a significant part of what I understood in my own process of getting well. Reverse Therapy really is working on the principle that all of our symptoms are based on a failure to respond to something emotionally, and that the symptoms are the body's way of bringing our attention to that in order that we can resolve it.

Again, it is a really good concept, and I think in some ways really useful. I think it is definitely PART of the picture, but like so many treatments out there it pitches itself as the whole solution, and in my experience that is not the case. Just like the Lightning Process, what it does is to ignore the other factors at play - so again, it says that there is nothing else physically going on, and that just correcting the emotional response will solve it all; and we have seen too many cases to believe that this can possibly be true for everyone - we are mind, body and emotions and it makes sense to address the issue at all levels - and that for some is going to be more significant than for others.

The other key issue with Reverse Therapy is that it seeks to deal with the emotional intelligence of the body and pretty much seems to ignore the mind and the anxiety. Well, people who have got to the point of M.E. and total burn-out are often very much in their heads and NOT very connected, like we have said. So even though ultimately, the ability to reconnect to the body's wisdom is a very key part of the healing process, for many people this is extremely hard. We have seen a large number of people where the very process of trying to figure out what it is that their body is trying to say has become a SOURCE of anxiety! So I think it simplifies things again a little too much. It doesn't take into account the role of the mind and the stress state in the illness, and it doesn't necessarily take into account the fact that it's not always that easy to just instantaneously pick up on what's happening in your inner wisdom. It can take a while! In other words, again, you have to deal with the whole picture - the mind and anxiety patterns, the emotional patterns and issues and disconnection, and the physical imbalances, in order to have the best chance of success.

A: I know a lot of people with M.E. do things like Yoga and Meditation and find that really helpful as part of their recovery but maybe it's helpful but not a whole answer, maybe talk briefly around that as well.

An: I'm a big fan of both. If we look at everything we've been talking about - being in touch with your body and getting into a healing state, learning how to understand and listen to yourself differently - both meditation and yoga facilitate that and are fantastic tools. But, if I use me as an example, I got to the point when I was trying to get better by meditating up to four hours a day, and it came to the point where I realised as long as I was in meditation I would be fine, but as soon as I hit the real world, things were not going as well! So, I think the problem is that meditation takes you to a good state (as does yoga), and over time it also teaches you to be there more, but it doesn't necessarily deal with the underlying stress patterns that are there, and the emotional patterns that are there in our relationship with the world around us. I think these are really great tools, and we absolutely stress their importance in recovery, but you need more than these in general, to heal fully.

A: OK, we've talked about quite a lot of different approaches, different ideas around the mind, the body, the emotions and so on, maybe at this point we could break it down to a few specifics and key points people can focus on?

An: Absolutely. I would say the first key thing is that very often, as we've said, we're in a stress state when we have M.E., and that is usually a combination of factors, but a significant proportion of that is to do with the fear that is there around the illness. Which is completely logical by the way; it's completely logical if you've gone through something quite horrible you're going to want to avoid doing it again, so we start to limit and get scared of the world around us. Whether it's foods that could make us ill, or doing things that could make us ill, we start to develop a lot of fear and anxiety.

So the first thing to do really is to begin to learn, or rather un-learn, the patterns we've learnt of stress and fear that are usually going on in fairly significant ways. Very often also it's useful to say that that isn't just about the illness. There are usually anxiety patterns that very much pre-dated getting ill.

A: So you are saying that there is the psychology side prior to M.E., and there's a psychology side resulting from someone having the illness.

An: Exactly that. And in a way, very often what the illness does is feed the patterns that were there before we got ill. So if we were a worrier anyway, suddenly we have a lot to worry about! So that's one of the key things to begin to work with and begin to resolve, because while that's there, it's blocking everything else from improving.

A: As we were saying earlier, people are in almost the opposite state to what they need to be in, in order to be able to heal. There's a state of stress, a state of healing and they're in a state of stress.

An: And actually we have more control over what is happening in our bodies physically than we might know, through working with our psychology. I know that can be challenging, because it feels like it is just happening to us, but when you begin to understand the real links between what happens in your mind and your thoughts and your emotions, and what then happens physically, there are very strong correlations. I was saying to a patient the other day, that although it feels random, in fact, often the symptoms and state you are in on any day is not just 'happening' and out of your control. There are, if you like, certain 'ingredients' that go into creating that situation - that physical 'state' - and those ingredients consist of a whole host of factors: what you are thinking (so the messages you are sending your body, how you are telling it to chemically react - whether that is a stress or a healing state); the emotions that are happening and have been happening for you; what you have physically been doing and the state you have been in whilst you were doing it; whether you are giving your body what it needs in terms of nutrients, movement, even fun! If you put certain things into a cake you're going to get the same cake out every time, and actually the more we begin to understand and really be clear about what is happening in our psychology and in our emotions, the more we begin to understand how we are getting the results that we are getting.

A: Good, so the first thing is dealing with the state of being in stress, and you talked about the emotional side of it as well.

An: Yes, I think that's really relevant for a lot of people. I think there are strong emotional background patterns and issues going on around the illness. One thing that's fascinated me is how much relationship there is between stored emotion - so emotion we haven't been able to contact or express - and symptoms such as pain in the body.

A: And that's interesting as well with people with Fibromyalgia, because pain is the main thing that differentiates Fibromyalgia from M.E. and Chronic Fatigue Syndrome.

An: Yes. I have been fascinated with this over the time that I've worked in this field, and there genuinely seems to be a strong link between physical pain and undigested emotional pain. Most people, by the time they've burnt out, have a fair bit of emotionally held 'stuff'.

A: Yes, I remember someone once said that things that are not being expressed emotionally have to go somewhere, and often physical pain can be the expression of things that are not being emotionally expressed.

An: I think that's true. Maybe it sounds a little 'out there' to some people, but the more that we work with it, the more we can see that this actually does seem to be the case. And we've had lots of clients work through their physical pain symptoms by working emotionally with what's happening, with techniques like Emotional Freedom Technique

255

which is one of the tool kits we use. So, it can make a massive difference to physical symptoms.

The other thing to say is that for a lot of people there are emotional contents to the way they're physically feeling. And we can see that if we start to look at the words that we use, so when we're tired, we're actually 'exhausted' or 'drained', and drained could describe something emotional or it could describe something physical. Those kinds of descriptions give us a bit of a clue that very often a physical state that we're in has emotional background content to it as well. There are different kinds of tiredness, different kinds of fatigue, and there is a fatigue that is quite significantly emotionally driven, where we just feel heavy and drained and emotionally exhausted.

A: Yes, and I think the thing is for people maybe that are watching this, and thinking, "This just sounds a bit too much for me and is a bit too radical," The thing I always say is that, "We may not like it, and it may not be the way we want it to be, but it is what it is." And, I know that I was hugely resistant to the role of psychology in my illness when I had M.E., but the point that I stopped resisting it and said, "Well, you know what, let's explore this, maybe it is true," that's when something new opened up for me.

An: I think that's really true. One of the key things that I find as a massive factor in recovery tends to be people having the attitude of curiosity and real openness to try things. I was the same as you, I would have laughed in your face if you'd said some of this, and it's only really the experience of having gone through it both personally, and as a practitioner, that I've really learnt to see the potential of the body, and to see the complexity of the system.

We are so arrogant to assume we understand how everything works, and that the body is a simple machine that just needs fixing. Actually there is massive complexity to the body, to the mind, to this system - energetically and emotionally and in every way, so we have to be open to it. Because the reality is, traditional medical models don't work for most people dealing with C.F.S., M.E. and Fibromyalgia, which means that we have to look elsewhere for solutions.

I think perhaps it's also worth saying that what makes the model of treatment we use at the clinic so unique is the integration of so many different approaches. Because of our immense experience of all the different treatments out there, we are able to pull together the best of all of them and help each patient create their own individual roadmap for their journey to recovery. This generally saves patients a lot trial and error, and ultimately money, from trying all the different things on their own.

A: We've got about three to four minutes left, and I was just thinking that we've talked about the role of psychology in actually treating the illness and recovery, but I think there's also a role for people in terms of staying positive, staying inspired, staying motivated. What would you say about that for people that either are watching this and have M.E. or for people that are just interested from a life point of view who are going through something very difficult and want to keep that level of inspiration that things can change?

An: I think for a lot of people recovery is not a real smooth upwards curve. There are obstacles that get in the way, and that's part of the learning. So, staying inspired is really key. I think sometimes having other people around you who you can connect to, who understand what you're going through is pretty important. I find that a lot with our patients: saying it's so good to talk to someone who gets it.

I also think we need to listen to things that inspire us, watch things that inspire us, read things that inspire us, and support ourselves in remembering why we are working so hard to get well. And I think also being kind to yourself - having compassion for yourself and your process - is important. Sometimes we can really drive ourselves or expect certain things of ourselves and beat ourselves up when it's not going great. Be compassionate, you are learning. You wouldn't expect a toddler to learn how to walk instantaneously, and us trying to recover is a similar process. You've got to be patient with yourself and take the time to generally be nice to yourself in that process.

A: Good, and I'm also curious in the last few minutes, that you talked a little bit about that for you it was quite a gift in terms of how you changed and how your experience of the world changed, and I was curious a little bit that about what life is like for you now, now that you are recovered? When you look back on your journey, what's maybe one of the key lessons that you take from that?

An: I think one of the key lessons is to understand that what is happening is a journey that we can learn from, and I think the point when I began to see what was going on for me not just as something awful that had happened to me, but something I could use and learn from - and that would ultimately take me forwards and make me stronger - was the point when things began to turn around. Truthfully that's what I used to cling to and use, to move me forwards.

A: You know, it's like you described, you can be fully recovered from M.E., and yet the journey of life still continues...

An: Oh yeah!

A: ...and I think what is interesting listening to you speak is that it's almost like the M.E. experience triggered that journey, which has been a gift beyond just your recovery, because it's been a gift of a way of approaching and experiencing your life.

An: I say to people quite often that you're learning to be healthy, and that is an ongoing process, because you learn to be healthy to a point where you're physically healthy, but you're also learning how to be more and more of yourself, and that learning process just keeps going. So, it's the beginning of a journey for many people of understanding themselves at a much deeper level, a much more powerful level I think.

A: That's wonderful. Well thank you for your time today.

An: Thank you.

Introduction to CFS/ME and the
Integral Approach to Medicine

Introduction to CFS/ME and the Intergral Approach to Medicine
By Alex Howard and Niki Gratrix (August 2009)
Published in CAM Magazine September 2009

CFS/ME is still an illness that is regarded by orthodox medical circles as "puzzling" and with unknown aetiology. As any practitioner who has spent any time with CFS/ME patients can attest, they can confound, confuse and be downright difficult to treat with any real success. Understandable reasons exist for scepticism that the illness is even "real." No diagnostic markers exist. Standard biochemical blood tests all routinely come back normal. Also there are few observable clinical symptoms.

With no visible sign of illness, clinicians have to effectively be drawn inside the patient's internal experience and rely on reported feelings of bone-crushing fatigue, "brain-fog" and pain. Due to the conventional approach to medicine which tends to downplay, ignore and distrust internal subjective feelings and statements by patients, the medics wrongly concluded that if there was no physical objective evidence then the patient must be making it up! ME/CFS patients have thus had a rough ride with conventional medicine in the last 50 years.

We believe CFS/ME will become one of the most prevalent diseases of the 21st century. A report from the Department of Health Working Group (2002) summarised that approximately 0.2-0.4% of the population suffer from CFS/ME (122,000-244,000 million people based on population estimates of UK as 61 million). Studies of CFS/ME patients in 1996 and 1997 confirmed patients have disability rates similar to multiple sclerosis, rheumatoid arthritis, lupus, heart disease, diabetes and other serious illnesses (Komaroff et al 1996, Buchwald et al 1996, Anderson et al 1997).

In response to this, in 1998 the Chief Medical Officer in the United Kingdom commissioned an independant CFS/ME Working Group to write a report on all aspects of the illness after stating, "I recognise chronic fatigue syndrome is a real entity. It is distressing, debilitating, and affects a very large number of people. It poses a significant challenge to the medical profession." (Department of Health Working Group Report 2002). Despite that statement, there are still conventional practitioners who do not accept this illness is real. This view is something that any person with the illness, treating the illness, or with family or friends suffering from it would assign to ignorance. Of those practitioners that believe the illness is real, there is no small amount of controversy around treatment protocols within both orthodox medical research, the CAM world and among sufferers.

Within orthodox circles there are groups which believe CFS/ME is a psychiatric illness. Other researchers and clinicians believe it is an immune system disorder; others say it is a low-grade viral or/bacterial infection or set of co-infections; others are linking it to a malfunction of the heart, blood hyper-coagulation, HPA axis imbalances and still others suggest at the core it is caused by mitochondrial dysfunction or a methylation cycle crash or block. In the CAM world there are camps stating the only treatments necessary are brief psychological therapies. Others believe structural anatomical imbalances in the spine or in the temporomandibular joint are at the core of the problem. Others focus on food intolerances, gut dysbiosis, toxicity and nutritional deficiencies. Still others believe energetic or spiritual healing can make a fundamental difference.

To successfully treat CFS/ME the very paradigms of medicine and the orthodox approach have to be challenged. No other illness we know of challenges so strongly the artificial schism that exists between mind and body mainly in Western approaches to healthcare. In addition the disease is challenging CAM practitioners to "up their game" if they are to make headway with these patients. And we must not forget the patients: when faced with this plethora of treatments, they are often overwhelmed, spend thousands on one treatment after another or end up doing nothing.

We believe there is a framework, an approach which effectively and elegantly resolves all of this controversy. CFS/ME is an illness that taught us as a clinic to approach treatment of chronic disease from a truly comprehensive framework or understanding of mind-body medicine. The philosophical model which underpins everything we do in the clinic is based on what's called the "Integral" approach to medicine. By Integral we mean it in the context of the work by Ken Wilber. ME/CFS lends itself very well as a case study to examine the Integral Approach in action.

Integral framework to Mind-Body medicine

Integral means "all inclusive" or leaving nothing out. This term is different from "integrative" medicine. The terms "holistic" or "integrative" are often vague and vary dramatically in meaning and practical application from practitioner to practitioner. The Integral Approach defines what we mean by being "holistic" in medicine. It means that we map the approach to health onto Wilber's 4 Quadrants - see the diagram overleaf.

This model came about through a lifetime study of reality - summarized in his book a "Brief History of Everything" -- by the American philosopher and teacher Ken Wilber. We encourage readers who want to understand more on the model to read this book, as there is a level of detail which is beyond the scope of this article.

The model states that all of reality consists of a holon - a "whole that is part of other wholes" -- and all of existence or experience can be classified into Four Quadrants by differentiating between the external objective world (two right Quadrants) and the subjective world of inner beliefs and attitudes (left two Quadrants). Further categorization can then be made between the collective internal and the collective external (bottom two Quadrants). When applying this to the health of an individual we now have a map of all possible factors that can affect and influence human health.

Four Quadrant approach to medicine

Internal Subjective - Individual	External Objective – Individual
• Meaning • Thoughts, beliefs, attitudes • Emotions, feelings • 5 senses – see, touch, hear, taste, smell	• Popp's biophoton field • Physics of the energy body • Biochemistry and structural mechanics • Atoms, molecules, organs, systems, the body "electric"
Internal Intersubjective Group - Cultural	External Interobjective Group – Social
• Relationship between patient and physician • Support and understanding from friends, family • Cultural understanding and beliefs around the illness, predjudices • Cultural beliefs around treatment modalities	• Financial support from the NHS • Financial support through insurance companies • Environmental toxins- pesticides, chemicals and electrosmog • Access to information - internet

Within each Quadrant there are also levels of treatment which will be explained in more detail below. For now it is useful to understand that conventional medicine exists almost entirely in the upper right Quadrant. It deals with the physical organism using purely physical interventions: surgery, drugs, medication and behavioural modification. Conventional medicine essentially believes in the physical causes of illness and therefore prescribes mostly physical treatments.

But the Integral model claims that every physical event must have 4 dimensions, therefore the top right Quadrant is but one fourth of the cause. The study of psychneuroimmunology has for example made it quite clear that a person's interior states play a crucial role both in the cause AND treatment of many illnesses. In addition to this, no human exists in a vacuum. Humans live in a cultural and social environment which they are intimately linked to and affected by. An Integral Approach to treatment therefore takes account of environmental factors, other social and cultural influences, as well as the internal beliefs values and attitudes of the patient

The point of Integral is not that we throw out conventional medical approaches; there is a fundamental time and place for conventional medicine. If you have an accident and break a leg you thank the paramedics and surgeons - we don't exactly care about your diet at that point! The point is the Integral Approach is more successful because you touch all bases. The aim is to take into account and integrate all Quadrants and levels within Quadrants - and not to ignore, downplay or rule out anything that there is to offer in each Quadrant.

Impact on the orthodox view of CFS/ME

When we look at health from the 4 Quadrant Integral Approach, it is like refocusing the camera lens and zooming right out. This is a far cry from orthodox medicine where we zoom in purely to the top right Quadrant. Beyond this there is further reductionism in conventional medicine - leading practitioners into specialization. Hence the human body is segmented into biological systems: immune, nervous endocrine and so on.

As a result, in the orthodox approach specialization leads to learning more and more about less and less.

Solutions to problems are often not found at the same level of thinking that created them. When orthodox practitioners come from this reductionistic approach it is no wonder an illness like CFS/ME "mystifies" them. Almost every scientific paper states CFS/ME

263

currently has an "unknown" aetiology. It's not until the treatment approach matches the location of the illness that results can be found.

Mind-body researchers like Dr Candace Pert, author of "Molecules of Emotion", have even gone beyond stating that previously segmented biological systems are interconnected. Pert and her colleagues now say that biological systems are part of an inseparable dynamic mind-body system, and mind and body has a bi-directional connection - meaning that a healing impulse from EITHER the physical or the psycho-emotional side can lead to correction of the entire system.

The foundation of the model takes a world view which challenges the basic assumption of orthodox medicine and this is why conventional medicine fails so miserably to treat a chronic multifactorial illness like ME/CFS. Conventional medicine purely assumes that matter came about before consciousness - therefore consciousness (mind and beliefs) do not cause physical changes in the body. However the 4 Quadrant model clearly does support the idea that mind and emotions DO affect the physical body.

The placebo effect is one of the most important proofs that the internal subjective impacts physicality. The typical view is that the placebo affect should be controlled or eliminated from studies, yet this phenomenon is a powerful proof of the link between intention or belief and physical bodily response. No agent in history has been more tested than the placebo!

Conventional medicine downplays influence of the impact of environmental toxins and cultural and social aspects while placing too much emphasis on the importance of, for example, genetics. Books such as "What it Means to be 95% Chimpanzee: Apes, People, and their Genes" by Johnathan Marks, PhD, and the work of cell biologist Bruce Lipton, PhD, address this issue head on.

Relevance to CAM practitioners

Many CAM practitioners are familiar with the limitations of conventional medicine.

We believe, however, that there are also insights for many CAM practitioners using this model. Many practitioners treating CFS/ME think they are "holistic" and are treating the whole person because they are using non-drug based treatments, are aware of environmental toxins and care about the psychological welfare of patient. If conventional medicine treats the illness, alternative treats the person.

However, many CAM practitioners we see get caught out on a number of factors:

1. They become overly focused on the top right or left Quadrant. So for example rather than drugs they are using herbs, or nutritional supplements. It's easy to simply replace drugs with natural alternatives but get caught up in an orthodox approach - rather than a drug pill for every ill, we use herbs or nutrition to treat symptoms rather than true causes.

On the other hand we note that some practitioners working in the top left hand Quadrant believe that mind and emotions - intentionality - creates everything. This is the "law of attraction" brigade or "thoughts create reality". Here the influence of environmental toxins or biochemical deficiencies are downplayed or ignored completely, often at the expense of patient welfare.

2. In addition to getting stuck in one Quadrant, CAM practitioners can also get stuck at one level of treatment within a Quadrant. Multiple levels exist in each Quadrant. This pyramid represents the top two Quadrants of the individual:

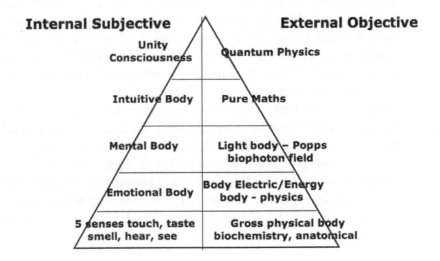

So for example a practitioner can get stuck only looking at biochemistry of the body or anatomical structure. The model suggests these practitioners might also consider the physics of the body. It is noticeable that in the UK and the US, there is a great deal of focus at the biochemistry and structural level, where as in parts of continental Europe, especially Germany, there is much more emphasis on treatment relating to "physics" of the body - the affect of geopathic stress, "electrosmog" and the "body Electric" with use of EAV, MORA, microcurrent therapies and so on.

On the upper left Quadrant, practitioners can also get stuck just treating the mental level with techniques related to NLP, while ignoring other therapies that deal better with emotional trauma, for example.

3. Just as the 4 Quadrant model asks conventional medics to start to acknowledge the importance and honour the internal subjective experiences of the patient, the model also demands that we do not throw out or ignore crucial elements of the upper right hand Quadrant - in particular the need for objective evidence-based medicine. We believe more CAM practitioners need to get involved with trials to prove the efficacy of their work, just as we suggest orthodox medics open their minds to all 4 Quadrants.

Four Quadrant approach applied to CFS/ME
When we apply the 4 Quadrant Model to ME/CFS we start to be able to understand and categorize all the treatments that are available out there. We start to see that each treatment is addressing a particular cause in a particular Quadrant - but it is not THE only or necessarily the most important factor for a patient - it may be just one-fourth of the story; less if the treatment is also just at one level within a Quadrant. We can start to understand how treatments relate to one another and the use of this model helps us to more quickly navigate a patient through the illness - ensuring we "touch all bases" of possible treatments.

It also helps us to more clearly start defining the fact that in the current definition of CFS/ME there are subgroups of patients where there are consistent specific patterns of illness showing up across the 4 Quadrants - although ultimately every single person's illness is unique.

Application to CFS/ME	Application to CFS/ME

• Energy-depleting personality types:
  o achiever type
  o anxiety type
  o helper type
  o trauma type
• Maladaptive stress response to illness
• Unresolved emotional trauma
• Diseases of the soul – crisis of meaning
	• Endocrine – thyroid, adrenal, pituitary
	• Immune dysfunction and toxicity
	• Metabolic imbalances – mitochondrial, malabsorption, leaky gut, dysbisois, food intolerances
	• Infections – viral, bacterial
	• Structural imbalances – spinal imbalances, turbomandibular joint problems, scar tissue
	• "Sensitivity to eletrosmog"
	• Genetics – methylation cycle polymorphisms
	• Cognitive behavioural therapy
	• SSRIs, sleep medications

Application to CFS/ME • Cultural Stigma of the illness as "unreal" • Lack of understanding from family, work, friends • Poor relations between doctor and patient	**Application to CFS/ME** • NICE guidelines and NHS treatment generally unhelpful • CAM therapy not covered by insurance

The model directly helps us start to identify where the location of the illness is. So as practitioners we are asking such questions as:

• Is the illness due to genetic polymorphisms in the methylation cycle? (Upper right Quadrant)
• Is there illness because the patient has what we call an "energy-depleting personality type" - one example is the chronic over-achiever? (Upper left Quadrant)
• Is it because they were unknowingly exposed to a large dose of pesticides for years because they lived next door to a farm? (Lower right Quadrant)
• Or was it because the patient grew up with an alcoholic father, an absent mother and then became ill, and the illness was perpetuated due to lack of cultural belief, support and understanding? (Lower left Quadrant)

How OHC addresses all Quadrants and all levels
In our experience patients often have a combination of causes from all Quadrants. There may be a fast or slow onset of the illness. Notably fast onset can be caused by a trigger originating from any of the 4 Quadrants - say a divorce, environmental exposure or a virus - but

there will have been long-term predisposing factors usually from all Quadrants in the run up to the illness.

We use the Enneagram system of 9 personality types to assess all patients who come into the clinic. There is very clearly a subgroup of CFS/ME who have certain personality characteristics such as being "achievers" and "helpers." A major component for a number of patients is also the "Maladaptive Stress Response": they find themselves locked in as a reaction to suffering from an illness for which there is so little understanding and that can feel like a life sentence of uncertainty and at times unbearable symptoms.

Just as it is possible to get stuck in the biochemistry only level and ignore the "body electric" in the upper right, so too do practitioners get caught in treating purely the mental aspects of the illness, missing out on treating the emotional aspects. That's why it is so important for us as a clinic to have developed a vast protocol of all the different components involved in ME, and also a strong referral network for areas we do not cover in house.

One important point we note here is that there are many excellent specialist practitioners in the US treating CFS/ME who take a very Integral Approach in general - however there is a conspicuous lack of treatment in the upper left Quadrant. The use of psychological techniques has not taken off like it has in the UK. This may be because practitioners have rightly been put off by looking at the weak positive results that Cognitive Behavioural Therapy (CBT) has in the treatment of CFS/ME.

In our experience, CBT is some 50 years out of date. Certain techniques known as "brief psychological therapies" -- such as EFT, NLP, EMDR and more -- are profoundly successful with subgroups of CFS/ME patients. This is especially true where the practitioners specialise in using these purely for ME patients. There are now some highly skilled practitioners in the UK - often they have suffered from the illness themselves and discovered these treatments worked so well they went on to become practitioners themselves.

Fundamentally important is also the lower left - cultural beliefs. Stigma around the illness and lack of understanding in our experience directly reduces a patient's expectation of recovery and creates stress. We have patients tell us stories like friends being diagnosed with cancer at the same time as they were diagnosed with CFS/ME and noticing the level of understanding, support and sympathy available with a clear, accepted illness. The friend would tell them they were happier to have been diagnosed with bowel cancer than go through what they would face with a diagnosis of CFS/ME.

Just a couple of ways we have worked to overcome this is by last year launching a social networking website specifically for patients of the clinic, so they can interact with others on a healing journey anywhere in the world, with a shared attitude that "recovery is possible." (see www.OptimumHealthCommunity.com)

We additionally have a bi-weekly series of conference calls, where patients have ongoing access to inspirational recovery stories, and the very latest ideas and techniques (see www.SecretsToRecovery.com)

To focus in the area of the lower right, as before mentioned, we feel that clinical trials are an essential ingredient to get access to increased government support and funding for illnesses such as ME. Beyond even our own two-year study, we have also set up a research charity to raise funds for further projects.

We have also recently been approached by several major insurance companies who are now funding treatment at the clinic, despite the fact that what we are doing is still, in the eyes of science, unproven. They are doing this because the sooner high-earning employees get back to work, the less they end up paying out, and they have seen a number of people get back to work using our protocols where patients were paying. These developments in the lower right are so important to over time increase the research base on effective treatments, and so enable access to them for more people. The reality is that it would ultimately cost the government less to fund more effective treatments, than be paying out the fortune it is each year on benefits for those affected by ME.

The practitioner changes first

The Integral Approach does not suggest practitioners train and become experts in everything or even just, say, naturopathy and transpersonal psychology. It suggests that they become "Integrally Informed" practitioners - which means they have a framework of understanding and appreciation for ALL factors which can be affecting a patient's health, so the practitioner would know how they fit into the wider picture and so they can know the strength and limitations of their own modality.

Ironically an Integral Approach to health means us as practitioners change first before we can change the lives of our patients. As such it is not about what the practitioner practises nor his/her modality of treatment - it is the awareness of the practitioner that counts.

In our experience when an approach like the 4 Quadrant theory is used to take account of the width and the depth of all causes of a chronic illness like ME/CFS, solutions and answers are reached faster and more effectively. Instead of looking for reductionistic complex biochemical problems to try to answer every problem, as an Integral practitioner you start to learn that actually all that is required is a "back to basics" approach in the upper right hand Quadrant.

In each Quadrant and level there are so many solutions available and applicable to patients that we are constantly looking to distil the "difference that makes the difference" for patients in each area. The challenge now at our clinic is to start to document and identify subgroups of CFS/ME patients, and also speed up our ability to identify where each person's illness location lies within the Quadrants and levels.

For the last five years we at the clinic have applied CANI - Constant and Never Ending Improvement -- to our treatment protocols for CFS/ME (and in fact every area of the clinics operations). This has forced us to constantly look bigger and wider, overcoming our own egos and often submitting to the realization that as a clinic with a psychology and a nutrition or physically focused division, together we are far greater than the sum of our parts.

Meglomania bred of isolationism: partial truths in the CFS/ME world

ME/CFS is a powerful case study for the Integral Approach to mind-body medicine. The CFS/ME world is beset with reductionistic theories, with practitioners as well as educated patients who claim to have "the" answer to the illness. These claims border on megalomania bred from so many practitioners working in isolation. And we echo Wilber's sentiments when he states "Nobody is smart enough to be wrong all the time." No human mind can be wrong 100% of the time.

We believe all specialists treating CFS/ME are honest, genuine people looking for answers to this illness. Thus all these practitioners have something important to say which we all need to take heed of. There are some extremely gifted scientists, researchers and clinicians in the CFS/ME arena who we see are searching for the "beautiful theory" of CFS/ME. In most cases this involves searching the upper right hand Quadrant for a single unifying theory that can explain all the underlying symptoms elegantly and compellingly. Strong contenders at the moment are blocks in the methylation cycle, mitochondrial malfunction, heart malfunction, sub-optimally functioning hypothalamic-pituitary-adrenal axis, immunological abnormalities or low grade co-bacterial or viral infections.

Notably, all these theories entirely ignore the inner state of the patient, who they are, who they were and how they experience their illness and whether they expect to recover or not. The physically-focused practitioners at our clinic are always humbled when they attend The 90-Day Programme offered at the clinic. To see a highly skilled psychologically-focused practitioner work magic with these patients is a constant reminder to avoid reductionistic thinking, and hence the reason our quartlerly cross-training seminars, integrated questionnaire and monitoring procedures are so vital as we train all the practitioners to be Integral Practitioners - not just nutritionists or psychology practitioners.

We say that a unifying single theory will never be found in a single Quadrant. We believe there IS a beautiful theory - and it is Integral theory. In our view is a time to invite conversation between practitioners specializing in treating CFS/ME. Practitioners who are not interested in speaking and learning from colleagues also treating the illness from different modalities will lose out - and so in turn will their patients. Patients themselves also need to understand that what may have worked for them is not necessarily going to be the truth and the way for many other patients with the same diagnosis - and Integral theory will tell them why.

For information on The Optimum Health Clinic's work with M.E., including ordering a free information pack (which includes the DVD documentary "Freedom From M.E.: Journeys to Recovery" mentioned by Alex in the chapter "My Journey with The Optimum Health Clinic" and the full version of the report "M.E. in the 21st Century") please visit:

www.FreedomFromME.co.uk

Call 0845 226 1762

Or write to:
The Optimum Health Clinic
Head Office and Training Centre
Bickerton House
25-27 Bickerton Road
London
N19 5JT

For information on Alex Howard's professional training courses in hypnotherapy, NLP, life coaching and ET, please visit:

www.consciouspsychology.com

To explore Alex's latest venture, a TV channel exploring awakening within daily life, please visit:

www.conscious2.com

If you would like to contact Alex directly, please e-mail:
whyme@TheOptimumHealthClinic.com

Books And Films

Stories of healing and the power of the human spirit:
Why I Survive AIDS (Niro Markoff Asistent)
The Journey (Brandon Bays)
Whose Hands are These? (Gene Egidio)
My Soul Purpose (Heidi von Heltz)
Close Encounters (Roxi Iain McNay)
The Way of the Peaceful Warrior (Dan Millman)
Mutant Message Down Under (Marlo Morgan)
Still Me (Christopher Reeve)
My Life and Vision (Meir Schneider)
The Healer (Jack Temple)
Grace and Grit (Ken Wilber)

Books to feed your mind (Easier reading):
SpeedReading (Tony Buzan)
The 7 Habits of Highly Effective People (Steven Covey)
You Can Heal Your Life (Louise Hay)
Feel The Fear and Do It Anyway (Susan Jeffers)
Self Matters (Phil McGraw)
Everyday Enlightenment (Dan Millman)
Awaken the Giant Within (Anthony Robbins)
Unlimited Power (Anthony Robbins)
Soul Without Shame (Byron Brown)
The Biology of Belief (Bruce Lipton)
Molecules of Emotion (Candace Pert)

Books to feed your mind (More challenging):
Core Transformation (Connirae and Tamara Andreas)
Change Your Mind and Keep the Change (Steve and Connirae Andreas)
Tranceformations (Richard Bandler and John Grinder)
Frogs into Princes (Richard Bandler and John Grinder)
Beliefs (Robert Dilts, Tim Halbom and Suzi Smith)
NLP and Health (Ian McDermott and Joseph O'Connor)
A Brief History of Everything (Ken Wilber)
Spiral Dynamics (Don Beck and Christopher Cowan)
Integral Spirituality (Ken Wilber)
Waking the Tiger (Peter Levine)

Books to heal your body (including suggestions from Niki Gratrix):
Quantum Healing (Deepak Chopra)
Unconditional Life (Deepak Chopra)
Age Power (Leslie Kenton)
Fast Food Nation (Eric Schlosser)
Detoxify or Die (Sherry Rogers)
Food is Better Medicine than Drugs (Patrick Holford and Gerome Burns)
The Sinatra Solution (Dr Sinatra)
Nourishing Traditions (Sally Fallon)
Total Health Cookbook and Program (Dr Mercola)
The Metabolic Typing Diet (William Wolcott)
Desperation Medicine (Ritchie Shoemaker)

Books to nourish your soul and spirit:
The Power of Now (Eckart Tolle)
A New Earth (Eckart Tolle)
Loving What Is (Byron Katie)
Diamond Heart - Books 1-4 (A. H. Almaas)
Essence (A. H. Almaas)
Illusions (Richard Bach)
Jonathan Livingston Seagull (Richard Bach)
One (Richard Bach)
The Return of the Rishi (Deepak Chopra)
The Knight in Rusty Armour (Robert Fisher)
The Spiritual Dimension of the Enneagram (Sandra Maitri)
The Link (Matthew Manning)
Anatomy of the Spirit (Caroline Myss)
The Celestine Prophecy (James Redfield)
Conversations with God: Books 1-3 (Neale Donald Walsch)
A Return to Love (Marianne Williamson)
Intimate Communion (David Deida)

Some films which have powerfully moved me:
8 Mile
Awakenings
City of Angels
Conversations with God
Dead Poets Society
Field of Dreams
Ghost
G. I. Jane
Gladiator
Lorenzo's Oil
Meet Joe Black
Message in a Bottle
October Sky
On a Clear Day
Patch Adams
Pay It Forward
Rain Man
Saving Private Ryan
Scent of a Woman
Tarzan
The Celestine Prophecy
The Cider House Rules
The Lion King
The Lord of the Rings
The Matrix
The Pursuit of Happiness
The Shawshank Redemption
The Sixth Sense
The Way of the Peaceful Warrior
Three Kings
Unbreakable
What the Bleep Do We Know?

Also available:

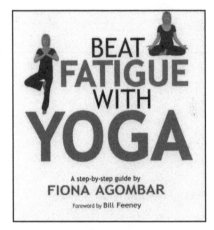

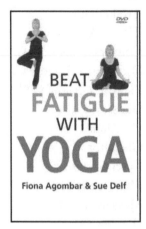

ISBN 1-901447-45-6
210 pages with illustrations

DVD   CRH 001

BEAT FATIGUE WITH YOGA (BOOK & DVD)
Fiona Agombar and Sue Delf

If you feel tired, drained or exhausted, it's likely yoga can help. Yoga is a complete integrated system for
healing and well being, and is the ideal, gentle way to address and gradually remove the causes of exhaustion.

'Beat Fatigue with Yoga' really is a unique DVD release. There are several DVDs available on yoga but most of them involve supermodels and perfect bodies. This DVD is for the ordinary person who gets tired; and that includes almost anyone. The programmes on this DVD are designed for people in different conditions. There is a section for those who have Chronic Fatigue Syndrome and thus have severely compromised energy; and there are other sections for those who just get tired sometimes after a busy day. The DVD is thus designed to be used by people of all abilities, with postures deliberately chosen to help them relax and increase their levels of health and vitality.

The DVD features Sue Delf, one of the UK's most experienced yoga teachers who teaches at the famous TRIYOGA centre in London and Fiona Agombar, author of the well known book also titled "Beat Fatigue with Yoga." Both have gentle and encouraging style, perfect for those just starting doing yoga, and those who already have a practice.

There are also bonus section interviews with Fiona Agombar and Alex Howard (author of 'Why Me?') on their own journeys from Chronic Fatigue to recovery.

The Book or The DVD will show you how to:
- **Find easy ways to relax and improve your stamina**
- **Work out the causes of fatigue**
- **Balance your chakras, or personal energy centres**
- **Use breathing excercises to boost vitality**
- **Use simple yoga routines to increase energy and stretch and tone your physique**

"Fiona Agombar describes in her book how simple daily exercises can help rebuild your life."
Daily Express
"This book will help you work out the causes of your fatigue, boost your energy levels and tone your body." Good Housekeeping
"This book is brilliant - it really helped me." Jane Roscoe, Producer, BBC Radio 2

CONVERSATIONS ON NON-DUALITY
Twenty-Six Awakenings

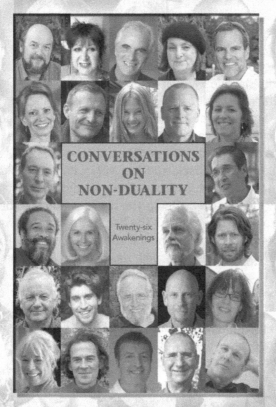

A fascinating compilation of interviews with twenty six
ordinary people, including many contemporary non-duality teachers,
all of whom have been through extraordinary
experiences leading to amazing new perceptions.

Available on from all good outlets

CONSCIOUS.TV

conscious.tv is a UK based TV channel broadcasting on the Internet at www.conscious.tv. Our programmes are also shown on channels broadcast via Sky and Freesat in the UK.

We aim to stimulate debate, question, enquire, inform, enlighten, encourage and inspire people in the areas of Consciousness, Science, Non-Duality and Spirituality. We have made over 300 programmes and record new interviews on a regular basis.

We welcome any feedback and are very interested in suggested topics and guests for future programmes so drop us a line on info@ conscious.tv if you have anything you would like to feed back to us.

We have two email newsletters. The first is a general Newsletter that we send out every 3 months and the second is our 'New Programme Alert list' which means you will be notified every time a new programme is available to watch on the channel. Email us on info@ conscious.tv if you would like to be included on either or both of these.

Many of our programmes are also available as audio only downloads and others can be viewed as transcripts.

Do go to www.conscious.tv and discover our world.....

www.conscious.tv